PRAISE FOR

Healing Words for the Body, Mind and Spirit

■

"*Healing Words for the Body, Mind and Spirit* is written beautifully, and in such a way that we can truly understand how to use the magic and power of words to transform our lives."

SANDRA INGERMAN, author of

Medicine for the Earth and *Soul Retrieval*

⌒

"What a helpful and readable book, full of wisdom. Ponder these pages, for Caren Goldman's *Healing Words* offers a wealth of anecdotes, reflections, and stories that give fresh energy and insight for the spiritual journey."

MARGARET BULLITT-JONAS,

author of *Holy Hunger*

⌒

"Caren Goldman invites us to participate in healing on any or every level of our being. The goal is nothing short of embracing life fully. A skillful and clear writer, Caren is also a sensitive and compassionate guide who speaks heartfully and wisely—from her own experience of the ten thousand joys and ten thousand sorrows we all face as human beings."

MIRKA KNASTER, author of

Discovering the Body's Wisdom

"This is an inspirational, enriching, sensitive guide for anyone facing a difficult time. Caren Goldman's unique insights, thought-provoking ideas, and practical ways to approach life will inspire her readers. She writes with wisdom and heart and gives her readers a wonderful journey through healing."

ELISE NEEDELL BABCOCK, author of
When Life Becomes Precious

"The power of language never ceases to amaze me. Caren Goldman shines a healing light of new understanding and clarity on how we can approach language with intention and transform our bodies and spirits in the process. A truly remarkable book."

JENNIFER LOUDEN, author of *The Woman's Comfort Book*
and *The Comfort Queen's Guide to Life*

"An inspired idea whose time has come. A great way to overcome the hopelessness and helplessness of the many mind-boggling illnesses that plague our society today. Caren offers us a positive transformative experience that can lead to a whole new definition of healing. Every writer, every reader, every speaker knows that words hold power—it's time for all of us to allow their power to heal us, not just instruct or entertain. It is a much-needed book."

JANE VOORHEES, recipient of the Charles Haslom Award for
Excellence in Bookselling and co-owner of Malaprops Bookstore,
Asheville, North Carolina, *Publishers Weekly* Bookseller of the Year (2000)

"Caren Goldman is making it possible to take a thoughtful journey inward and achieve a quality in life we all desire. Guides and mentors are a great blessing, and Caren is just that for this reader."

EMOKE B'RACZ, past president of the
South Eastern Booksellers' Association (SEBA)

HEALING
WORDS

for the Body, Mind and Spirit

■

101 WORDS
TO INSPIRE AND AFFIRM

CAREN GOLDMAN

Foreword by
BELLERUTH NAPARSTEK

MARLOWE & COMPANY
NEW YORK

Published by
Marlowe & Company
An Imprint of Avalon Publishing Group Incorporated
161 William Street, 16th Floor
New York, NY 10038

Library of Congress Cataloging-in-Publication Data
Goldman, Caren.
    Healing words for the body, mind, and spirit: 101 words to
inspire and affirm/by Caren Goldman.
        p. cm.
    ISBN 1-56924-585-1
    1. Spiritual healing—Meditations. I. Title.
    BL65.M4 G65 2001
    291.3'1—dc21

                                            2001030023

                9 8 7 6 5 4 3

Designed by *Pauline Neuwirth, Neuwirth & Associates, Inc.*

Printed in the United States of America
Distributed by Publishers Group West

In loving memory of
Muriel Harriet Oglesby and Edwin Henderson Voorhees

A PORTION OF THE PROCEEDS OF THIS BOOK
WILL BE DONATED TO BREAST CANCER RESEARCH

Contents

■

Foreword

BY BELLERUTH NAPARSTEK

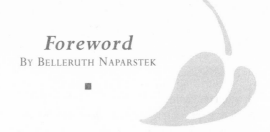

GETTING DIAGNOSED WITH a life-changing or life-threatening illness presents such a confusing rush of odd, contradictory reactions. Sitting in my therapist's chair for over thirty years, I've been afforded a powerful look into the fear, grief, elation, shame, relief, and anger that gets turned loose inside a person's weary, shell-shocked body when confronted with bad news.

We all carry a basic, narcissistic belief that it can't happen to us. This is how we get through the arbitrary dangers of the day, after all—by assuming we are cloaked in magical protection that renders us immune from the ugliness and bad fortune we see landing on others.

And because we cherish our fantasy that we are in control of our lives—especially dear to us citizens of the West—we tend to believe that our luck has been earned, through good character and smart choices.

So the news of illness catalyzes a disorienting undoing of some of our most closely held assumptions about ourselves and our lives. Like Alice, we fall topsy-turvy down the rabbit hole and land, naked and trembling, in an entirely new place. It's weird territory, where the old rules and definitions simply don't apply. Strange and scary as it is, though, it's also exciting, life-changing and god-awful interesting.

If we're lucky, our painful circumstances become a riveting invitation for growth and spiritual awakening on a newer, deeper level. As with all undoings, we've been handed an opportunity to reexamine and recreate ourselves, to reaffirm or redefine our sense of meaning and purpose. Any artist knows that deconstruction has its payoffs, and we are, of course, the artists of our lives.

Caren Goldman, who has surely earned her stripes with decades of brilliant writing about psychospiritual matters, has gone the extra mile here, by taking the battering force of a stunning configuration of family illnesses—her own and those dearest to her—and turning it into this wonderful book.

Working with *Healing Words* can make order out of chaos and provide just enough structure to return a sense of control, hope, and efficacy to someone whose life has been pulled out from under him. It's designed to be used in whatever dosage the reader is up for—word by word, page by page.

It's just enough gentle, wise guidance to open up safe footing and clearly lit choices on a trail that must be traveled, one way or the other. With my dear and trusted friend Caren, I can promise you this: you'll always get the high road. Blessings on your journey.

Belleruth Naparstek
Cleveland Heights, Ohio
May 18, 2000

Belleruth Naparstek is the author of *Staying Well with Guided Imagery*, *Your Sixth Sense* and the *Health Journeys Guided Imagery* audiotapes.

Introduction

∎

I MET THE MUSE that inspired me to write *Healing Words for the Body, Mind and Spirit* during the fall of 1999. She appeared when my husband, Ted, and I faced one health-related crisis after another. First, my mother fell and underwent hip replacement surgery. Just ten days later, my father-in-law died of congestive heart failure. Upon returning from his funeral, I received word from my doctor that a lump I had found on my breast was malignant. Then, a month after my surgeon removed the small cancer from my left breast, my mother returned to the hospital. She went to have a pacemaker inserted in her chest—a simple procedure. However, during preop testing, her radiologist discovered a malignant mass in her lung. Fortunately, it was contained and operable. Unfortunately, at the same time, our thirty-one-year-old daughter, Jamie, learned she had multiple sclerosis. While we were absorbing the impact of that blow, my sister delivered yet another: "Mom's had a heart attack. It doesn't look good," she said. "You'd better get down here." Six days later, almost six months after she shattered her hip, my mother died as my two sisters and I sat by her bedside.

ON THE DAY that my muse visited for the first time, Ted and I had decided to declare a "snow day" in the midst of the emotional chaos we felt inside and an Indian summer that warmed the autumn air outside. Tired of being wrapped in an unbroken chain of health-related phone calls and medical procedures, we canceled pending appointments, threw some bare essentials in the car, and headed for our small home in the wild and wonder-filled mountains of West Virginia.

While traveling the interstate highways and two-lane country roads leading to Berkana, our simple shelter nestled in a wildlife preserve, Ted and I shared our thoughts, feelings, pain, and plans. For hours, laughter, sadness, and tears erupted from a deep well of emotions. Sobs, sniffles, chuckles, chortles, ahas and uhs filled gaps in our banter until we both felt verbally exhausted and slipped into mutual silence. As Ted drove, I stared out my side window. Colorful leaves that blanketed the sunlit, windy world on the other side mesmerized me.

As quilted patches of tilled farmland melded into mountains covered with oak, maple, birch, and ash trees, I noticed that the dying leaves never took a nosedive straight to the ground. Instead, upon breaking from their boughs, they would ride currents of wind before landing. Sometimes, they'd look like gliders and sail lazily through the air. Other times, a gust would toss them back and forth, like riders on wild stallions circling a fenced-in corral. Occasionally, a whirlwind would catch them and they'd deftly spiral upward like Olympic ice skaters. Indeed, it seemed that no matter what path it was taking to the ground, each leaf was relishing the moment and its last opportunity to say "Yes!" to the life being left behind.

Delighted by the unrehearsed dance going on all around me, I found a passage from Deuteronomy bouncing around in my head to the beat of some nameless tune:

> I call heaven and earth to witness against you today that I have set before you life and death, blessings and curses. Choose life so that you and your descendants may live.

At first, the tune was interesting—calming. But, mere miles and many rounds later, I became really desperate for it to stop droning. Silently singing several verses of "Amazing Grace" in my head didn't work. Neither did the nursery rhymes, show tunes, patriotic songs, and popular ballads that I tried next. In fact, it didn't matter what I sang. Time after time, the monotonous tune I could not name prevailed, until, for no known reason, it stopped. Within seconds, an unfamiliar voice stepped in.

"Help others to find ways to help themselves heal," whispered a stranger inside my head. "Help others find ways to choose life—to say 'Yes!' "

With that said, her voice vanished.

Breaking the silence, I turned to Ted and said, "I think I just heard what's called a muse. She told me to do something to help others to help themselves. And as soon as I promised myself—or her—that I would, I saw an image of a book with a healing word written on each page."

WHEN WE RETURNED from West Virginia, Dr. Edgar Staren, M.D., Ph.D., director of the Cancer Institute at Medical College of Ohio, excised the small tumor from my breast and several lymph nodes from under my arm. Later, I awakened in the recovery room and found my surgeon and husband standing at my bedside. I could tell by their broad smiles that the cancer hadn't spread. Tears filled my eyes. Holding each of their hands in mine, I felt grateful and blessed.

In the days following my surgery, memories of the leaves and my promise to my muse resurfaced. Gradually, as images of the book that I had visualized in the car became more concrete, I began to see the word *healing* with new eyes. For over twenty-five years, I had written magazine articles about the remarkable power of words in the forms of prayer, affirmations, and meditation to support the healing process. Now, I realized that each word could be a stand-alone petition for healing in the way that a prayer, affirmation, or meditation was. Now, it was clear that these words, by themselves or combined, were oracles like Celtic runes or the *I Ching*—wise words that could gently and safely illuminate our journey towards physical, psychological, emotional, and/or spiritual healing.

What, you may wonder, is the healing path we take on such a journey? According to Larry Dossey, M.D., author of the groundbreaking books *Healing Words: The Power of Prayer and the Practice of Medicine* and *Reinventing Medicine*, "Genuine healing is frequently unexpected and radical, seemingly out of the blue, and often depends not on what we do or where we go but on how we choose to be." In other words, you don't have to be anywhere special to get on a healing path. Instead, your choices place you there.

What, you may wonder, does Dossey—or any one of us—mean by the word *healing*? There's no consensus. For example, to my mother's orthopedic surgeon, healing meant simply that the surgery to replace her hip was successful. Her bones mended, she tolerated rehabilitation well, and for a while she could walk and drive. Yet he told us that the fact that she felt terribly depressed weeks later had nothing to do with her recovery and was not his problem. For her cardiologist, healing meant that her condition would stop deteriorating and her heart could sustain her life without the medications and artificial life support that temporarily kept her alive.

However, for my surgeon, healing meant something more. His concerns were holistic. One week after my surgery, he not only reassured me that everything looked great and my prognosis for a cure was excellent, but he also wondered whether I might be interested in a support group or psychotherapy, and he affirmed using the complementary therapies I thought might facilitate my healing. He also asked Ted what he could do for him and reminded us that we could call him at home or the office anytime, because there were no "dumb" questions concerning my recovery and well-being.

Three physicians offering three different perspectives on the healing process—how many others, one wonders, might we hear from clergy, psychotherapists, philosophers, biologists, and the population at large?

Although most dictionaries don't define the words *healing* and *process* when they are linked, they do tell us that *healing* means to become whole and sound and return to health. But what, exactly, does it mean to become "whole?" Is it an attainable goal? Does that mean everything about me has to be perfect? That I have to be cured of an illness or infirmity? Or is it a process—a journey that teaches me how to embrace all the good and bad, broken and unbroken, perfect and imperfect, healthy and diseased parts of me? What, I wonder, would I have to do for those things to happen? What would it take for me to know with all my heart, mind, and soul that I have been healed and that I am whole? What might any of us have to do?

Perhaps the poet Mary Oliver struggled with similar questions when she wrote the poem "The Journey."

One day you finally knew
what you had to do, and began,
though the voices around you
kept shouting
their bad advice—
though the whole house
began to tremble
and you felt the old tug
at your ankles.
"Mend my life!"
each voice cried.
But you didn't stop.
You knew what you had to do,
though the wind pried
with its stiff fingers
at the very foundations—
though their melancholy
was terrible.
It was already late
enough, and a wild night,
and the road full of fallen
branches and stones.
But little by little,
as you left their voices behind,
the stars began to burn
through the sheets of clouds,
and there was a new voice,
which you slowly
recognized as your own,
that kept you company
as you strode deeper and deeper
into the world,
determined to do
the only thing you could do—
determined to save
the only life you could save.

■ ■ ■

I NOW INVITE you to use the healing words in this book to help guide you on your journey toward a greater appreciation of your potential for physical, emotional, psychological, and spiritual health and healing. Keep them close at hand. Give yourself permission to use them in whatever way works best for you. Experiment. For example, at first you may want to follow the suggestions below. Later, you might decide to come up with your own ideas. Or you may want to try your original ideas for using the words right away. Remember, there is no right or wrong way to use them, and you can change your mind at any time.

Here are some ideas to help you to get started:

1. Create a daily ritual that uses a word. Rituals help us to shift from ordinary time and space to sacred space. They can also help us clear our minds and focus on an intention for the well-being of ourselves and/or others. Begin your ritual by placing a candle or lantern on a personal altar or a table in your home. Then, as you light the wick or focus on the flame, state an intention in your own words. Your intention could be to listen carefully to whatever a healing word might say to you, no matter how foreign it might sound. Or your intention could be for someone else who is not present to discover the healing benefits of a word that you pick for them. After stating your intention, randomly pick a word. Allow time for it to evoke thoughts and images before reading the quotes and others' commentaries. You can also decide not to bother to look at what others have to say at all. The choice is yours.

2. Before going to bed for the night, pick a word. Focus on it and/or read what's written about it. Then write the word down on a piece of paper and place it under your pillow. Let the word dance before your mind's eye as you drift off to sleep. If the word speaks to you in a dream, take note of it. Keep a pad or tape recorder by your bedside so you don't have to get up.

3. Take time to journal about a word you've picked. Consider writing a poem about it, or "playing" it like the blues on a harmonica or a celestial harp or the black keys of a piano. Try expressing one or more healing words with any art materials you have on hand—markers, crayons, clay, paint, pastels, or just a pencil or a pen.

4. Walking or sitting with a word in a natural setting such as a park, garden, beach, forest, or desert can awaken dormant healing images in your psyche and soul. Additionally, if you find that a word suddenly inspires you to do something you wouldn't normally do—like baking a loaf of bread, telephoning someone, or going to sacred ground such as a church, synagogue, river, desert, or mountaintop—follow your nose, instincts, or intuition, and respect the fact that it may be a signpost leading you to a healing path.

5. Take this book with you when you go places. Pick a word and ponder it while stuck at a red light or put on hold. Try repeating the word you chose like a mantra as you drive somewhere or wait patiently for the party on the other end of the phone to answer your call. You might also pick a word when you get stuck waiting for an appointment in, of course, a waiting room.

6. Experiment with these words in group settings, too. When someone you know is suffering physically, emotionally, and/or spiritually, invite people to gather in a healing circle. It can be just for women, men, or both men and women. Create rituals for your time together that use *Healing Words* and other symbols of health, wholeness, and healing. These rituals can either come out of your religious and ethnic background or from other sources. For example, participants could listen to and/or move to music. There could be relevant readings from *Healing Words* and other sources of inspiration. A basket could be filled with words written on pieces of paper. Then each person could sing a word that they've picked and listen as the others in the circle sing it back. Or one word or a participant's name could be used like a mantra while everyone beats drums, shakes rattles, and takes turns smudging themselves or others with sweet grass and sage.

You get the idea. Unconditional offers of love, compassion and forgiveness for ourselves and others are not about dotting "I's" and crossing "T's," but matters of the heart and soul. When the intention is for healing, wholeness, and well-being, there are only "right" ways to use these words. So give your senses, imagination, and any muses whom you might hear permission to guide you. And finally, shift gears occasionally and see what happens if you take the position that you didn't pick the word—it picked you. If you do, consider these questions:

- Why this word at this time and in this place?
- What does this word mean to me?
- How have I experienced this word in my life?
- Where in my life might this word be missing?
- What can this word teach me about my healing process?

The quotes, affirmations, and text in the book can also help to expand your potential for self-healing. Maybe you will just look at a quote like a quote-of-the-day; maybe you will look at all three of the quotes at the top of the page and the two "wise old sayings" at the bottom and see whether one or more arrests your intention, or maybe you will decide to skip the quotes and go straight to the affirmation that uses your chosen word. In turn, you might take some time to either memorize it or to use it as a springboard to help you write an original affirmation that fits your circumstances and healing journey better.

The central text exploring each word varies. Sometimes it will be an anecdote about someone whose experience might resonate with yours and help you see an aspect of the healing process from a new perspective. Such stories might also stir you to creatively express yours in art, poetry, prose, movement or music. It may also be a timeless myth, or a sacred passage, or a poem, or some lyrics from a song that you're hearing for the first time or the hundredth. In fact, if you have heard or read some of the text before, try experiencing it with "new" eyes and ears and be open to doing that with your other senses and your heart as well. That way, whatever word you set before you will have a unique opportunity to speak to not only your mind and body, but your soul, too.

In her book *Close to the Bone*, psychiatrist and Jungian analyst Jean Shinoda Bolen reminds us that illness can initiate us into the soul realm. The word *liminal*, she explains, comes from the Latin word for *threshold*. When illness strikes, it often forces us to live at the edge—in the border realm between life and death. And this, she concludes, "is a liminal time and place."

Clearly, crossing any threshold can potentially initiate us into new ways of knowing the world. Just think about some that you have already crossed. You were born—thrust from the safe, soothing, connected world you knew in the womb into one in which you have had to be autonomous and seek shelter and significant connections. Once in this world, you crossed thresholds separating different stages of your life—some very consciously, some as a matter of course. For example, you left infancy and childhood behind for puberty, adolescence, adulthood, and, possibly, old age. Throughout your school years you crossed other thresholds as you made the transition from elementary school to high school and then to college, the work force, or the armed services. One day you lived in your parents' home, but the next day you didn't. You also straddled thresholds and crossed them when you fell in love or committed yourself to another or when a significant relationship ended. The same might be true for a job you started or one that ended. Indeed, Bolen tells us, whenever we are initiated into knowing something we did not know before on a body level, we cross a threshold. So it is with illness (and, I might add, remarkable recoveries) which, as Bolen says, "happens in and to the body and yet can profoundly affect the soul."

Healing Words speaks gently and persuasively to the thresholds we cross and the turmoil we feel in our minds, bodies, and souls when "dis-ease" strikes either us or those whom we care about and love. Take some time and recall such a moment in your life. Can you remember how out of control and anxious it made you feel? My daughter, Jamie, remembers feeling that way. Recently she told me that weeks after her doctor said the words "multiple sclerosis," she still felt as though her headlights were failing. They were dimming just when she needed them to shine their brightest to show her options and guide her through a maze of confusing information, thoughts, fears, and questions.

A closer look at the word *anxious* helps explain why any of us may have tunnel vision during times of physical, emotional, and spiritual crises. *Anxious* comes from the same family tree as the words *anguish*, *angst*, and *angina*. Furthermore, it is rooted in the Latin word *angere*, which means "to torment," and the Germanic *ang,* which means "compressed." How well we know that when disease—be it physical, mental, and/or spiritual—strikes, we feel both tormented and squeezed. Our breath may become shallow, our sleep may be disturbed, our appetite may wane, and our heart may feel as if a vise is gripping it or it's breaking. Subsequently, we find it difficult to see a wide range of choices. We begin to react to our experiences instead of responding to them, and our narrow focus makes our inner and outer worlds look dark and choiceless.

The words that follow on the pages of this book can help to safely illuminate the darkness that often prevails when we feel ill at ease, distressed, and/or out of control. Individually, each word is a pinpoint of light with a potential for enlightenment that can help us tap into a positive, natural healing power that is our birthright. Collectively, the words can function like a searchlight whose intense beam encircles a moonless night sky and penetrates the darkness.

In his book, *Man's Search for Meaning*, the renowned psychiatrist and Holocaust survivor Viktor E. Frankl wondered why some of the men who were imprisoned with him in Auschwitz and three other concentration camps not only survived their horrifying circumstances, but continued to grow in the process. "Man is ultimately self-determining," he concluded. "We must never forget that we may also find meaning in life even when confronted with a hopeless situation, when facing a fate that cannot be changed. For what then matters is to bear witness to the uniquely human potential at its best, which is to transform a personal tragedy into a triumph. . . . When we are no longer able to change a situation, we are challenged to change ourselves."

It is my hope that no matter what your situation, the words in this book will help support your desire to bring a healing quality to your mind, body, and spirit in loving, calming, and other positive ways. May they safely accompany you on whatever path you take to discover your hidden potential for wholeness as well as offer you new opportunities to choose to say "Yes!" to your life.

HEALING WORDS

for the Body, Mind and Spirit

ABUNDANCE

a great or plentiful amount;
fullness to overflowing

■

A man there was,
though some did count him mad,
The more he cast away,
The more he had.
JOHN BUNYAN

When we choose not to focus on what is missing from our lives but are
grateful for the abundance that's present . . . the wasteland of illusion
falls away and we experience Heaven on earth.
SARAH BAN BREATHNACH

Abundance is not a question of how much one has but of what one's
attitude is toward what one has. . . . The experience of abundance can-
not be found at the discursive or even at the emotional level. It must be
experienced within the body.
RICK JAROW

My HUSBAND, TED, is a minister in a large inner-city church. Whenever the subject of abundance comes up, he's apt to tell a story about a woman named Roslyn who visited on a Sunday when the Names Project AIDS Memorial Quilt was displayed in the church. Silently, as she sat before 16-foot sections of the tapestry that's helped millions of people to grieve the loss of friends, loved ones, and strangers who have died of AIDS, Roslyn seemed oblivious to the choir, clergy, and others who scurried around her.

That morning, Ted's sermon was about living out of abundance and sharing one's resources. "Our neighbors are having a very difficult time this year because of cold temperatures and welfare cuts," he said. "Daily, they knock on our doors for help."

After the service, Ted stopped to greet Roslyn, but she brushed him off. "I couldn't leave any money in the collection plate, but I did put in something else," she said before leaving. Moments later, an usher handed Roslyn's envelope to Ted. "This is all I have," the note inside began. "It is the last of what I received before getting a job. I'm sure that someone else needs them more than I do."

Enclosed were her food stamps.

Author Henry Miller tells us that the one desire that grows more and more is to give. "Giving and receiving are at bottom one thing, dependent upon whether one lives open or closed. Living openly one becomes a medium, a transmitter; living thus, as a river, one experiences life to the full, flows along with the current of life, and dies in order to live again as an ocean."

■

AFFIRMATION

I am grateful for the places where
I feel abundance in my life.

■

Riches are not from abundance of worldly goods,
but from a contented mind.
MOHAMMED

He who knows enough is enough will always have enough.
LAO-TZU

[3]

ACCEPTANCE

the act or process of accepting

■

Inside yourself or outside,
you never have to change what you see, only the way you see it.
THADDEUS GOLAS

You play the hand you're dealt. I think the game's worthwhile.
CHRISTOPHER REEVE

Never deny a diagnosis, but do deny the
negative verdict that may go with it.
NORMAN COUSINS

AN OLD ZEN story goes like this: An old Chinese farmer had a mare that broke through the fence and ran away. When his neighbors learned of it, they came to the farmer and said, "What bad luck this is. You don't have a horse during planting season." The farmer listened and then replied, "Bad luck, good luck. Who knows?"

A few days later, the mare returned with two stallions. When the neighbors learned of it, they visited the farmer. "You are now a rich man. What good fortune this is," they said. The farmer listened and again replied, "Good fortune, bad fortune. Who knows?"

Later that day, the farmer's only son was thrown from one of the stallions and broke his leg. When the neighbors heard about it, they came to the farmer. "It is planting season and now there is no one to help you," they said. "This is truly bad luck." The farmer listened, and once more he said, "Bad luck, good luck. Who knows?"

The very next day, the emperor's army rode into the town and conscripted the eldest son in every family. Only the farmer's son with his broken leg remained behind. Soon the neighbors arrived. Tearfully, they said,

"Yours is the only son who was not taken from his family and sent to war. What good fortune this is. . . . "

■

■

I dance to the tune that is played.
SPANISH PROVERB

You have to take it as it happens, but you should try to make it happen
the way you want to take it.
GERMAN PROVERB

ATONE

*to make amends or reparation for
an injury or wrong; to expiate.*

■

What is past is past,
there is a future left to all who have the energy to atone.
EDWARD G. BULWER

The beginning of atonement is the sense of its necessity.
LORD BYRON

The purpose of healing is to bring us in harmony with ourselves.
O. CARL SIMONTON

I FIND THE ARCHAIC definition of the word *atone* anything but outdated. Rooted in the Middle English word *atonen,* it once meant "to reconcile or harmonize" and had none of the breast-beating baggage the contemporary usage can carry. "To reconcile or harmonize"—how appropriate those words feel, since *atone* literally breaks down into two simple words—*at one.*

What does it mean to be "at one" with oneself, especially when we're ill or feeling ill at ease? If I know I am not "at one" because of hurts that I've caused another or acts I've committed that leave me uncomfortable, fragmented, or guilty, what must I do to heal those schisms?

Many years ago, Owen Ringwald told me a story that led me to a path of reconciliation. I met Owen at a human relations training workshop, where he was facilitating my group. Outside the workshop, we shared some meals and quiet walks and discovered we had many paths and friends in common. Months later, Owen and his wife, Mary, came to visit us in Ohio on their way from Delaware to their son Alan's home in Indiana.

The next morning, as we rocked back and forth on the swing on our porch, I asked Owen, then in his seventies, a question that I can't remember now. However, his answer changed my life. Owen began talking about Alan and said, "I had bypass surgery recently. Beforehand, Alan kept calling and insisting he wanted to fly in to be with me. 'It's not necessary,' I kept telling him. 'You don't have to be here.' But he persisted until I finally said, 'Alan, whatever the outcome, it will be okay. I love you, and I have no unfinished business with you.' "

Unfinished business. Why does unfinished business with another keep us from being "at one" with ourselves? What must we do to finish unfinished business with others—spouses, parents, children, relatives, friends, and adversaries both living and dead? Owen left later that day, and we never saw each other again. Yet, each time I tell his story, it reminds me that before I can know the healing that comes with being "at one" with myself, I must complete my unfinished business and be reconciled to others.

■

AFFIRMATION

More and more I'm aware of my unfinished business with others and myself.

■

On the day of atonement—you shall have the trumpet sounded
throughout all your land.
LEVITICUS 25:9

The hidden harmony is stronger than the visible.
HERACLITUS

ATTITUDE

a state of mind or a feeling; disposition;
a general cast of mind

■

Keep your face to the sunshine and you cannot see the shadows.
HELEN KELLER

We who lived in concentration camps can remember
the men who walked through the huts comforting others,
giving away their last piece of bread. They may have been few
in number, but they offer sufficient proof that everything can be taken
from a man but one thing: the last of the human freedoms—to choose
one's attitude in any given set of circumstances.
VICTOR FRANKL

Attitude is everything. Mae West lived into her eighties believing she
was twenty, and it never occurred to her that her arithmetic was lousy.
SOUNDINGS

WE OFTEN HEAR that attitude is everything and that it's important to have a positive one. However, for many people suffering from physical, emotional or spiritual *dis*ease, the call to have one overarching state of mind may be disheartening. Might we not feel more aligned with ourselves if we abandon the quest for one idealized attitude? That way we can give ourselves permission not only to hope for a positive outcome, but to have attitudes that are *gracious, kind, loving, upbeat, confident, forgiving, bitter, angry, melancholy, depressed, fearful, gloomy, pessimistic,* or even *horrible,* too. In the book *The Feminine Face of God*, Sherry Anderson and Patricia Hopkins write, "An attitude of 'not-knowing' can be like rain falling on the hard-packed soil of our lives. If we are willing, it can soften us, so we can feel gratitude and compassion and our own human vulnerability."

Author Dan Millman often tells the following story about the healing power of a courageous boy's willing and eager attitudes. According to Millman, there was a little girl in a California hospital who suffered from a rare, life-threatening disease. Her only chance of recovery depended upon a blood transfusion from her five-year-old brother. Miraculously, the boy had survived the same disease and now had the antibodies to combat it. The doctor explained the situation to the little boy and then asked him whether or not he would be willing to give his sister his blood. He only hesitated for a moment before taking a deep breath and saying, "Yes, I'll do it if it will save Liz."

During the transfusion, the boy lay in bed and smiled as the color returned to Liz's cheeks. Then his face grew pale. With a trembling voice he asked the doctor, "Will I start to die right away?" Being so young, he had misunderstood the doctor. He thought he was going to have to give his sister *all* of his blood.

■

AFFIRMATION

My willingness to acknowledge all my attitudes helps awaken
me to my potential to heal my wounds.

■

A clever person turns great troubles into little ones
and little ones into none at all.
CHINESE PROVERB

The dog that wags its tail won't be beaten.
JAPANESE PROVERB

AUTHENTIC

having a claimed and verifiable origin
or authorship

■

We all wear masks, and the time comes when we cannot remove them
without removing some of our own skin.
ANDRÉ BERTHIAUME

The striking thing about death, she thought, was its eventfulness.
It made you see you were leading a real life.
Real life at last! you could say.
ANNE TYLER

I'm tired of everlastingly being unnatural and never doing anything I
want to do. I'm tired of acting like I don't eat more than a bird, and
walking when I want to run and saying I feel faint after a waltz when I
could dance for two days and never get tired. . . . And I'm tired of pre-
tending I don't know anything, so men can tell me things and feel
important while they're doing it.
MARGARET MITCHELL

THOMAS MOORE, THE best-selling author of *Care of the Soul*, believes that
we suffer soul loss whenever we try to fit some norm of health or correctness instead of "living from the burning core of the heart, with the creativity that comes from allowing the soul to blossom in its own colors and shapes."

But how, one wonders, are we to live that way? First, Moore advises, we
must uncover our "original self," a process and potential that requires us to
live with both paradox and originality.

An "original self," he explains, is "one who came into this world full of
possibility and destined for joyful unveiling and manifestation. It is this per-

son we glimpse in another when we fall in love or when we idealize a leader or romanticize an artist. This is the person who comes to life in us briefly as we get married, start a course in school, or try on a new job—before worry and cynicism have set in."

To find this "seed of wondrous possibility that reeks with pleasure," Moore tells us that we must go far beneath the many thick layers of indoctrination about who we should be. Moreover, he says, "chronically trying to be someone other than this original self, persuaded that we are not adequate and should fit some norm of health or correctness, we may find a cool distance gradually separating us from that deep and eternal person, that God-given personality, and we may forget both who we were and who we might be."

Pablo Picasso put it this way: "My mother said to me, 'If you become a soldier, you'll be a general; if you become a monk you'll end up as the pope.' Instead, I became a painter and wound up as Picasso."

■

AFFIRMATION

When I peel back the layers covering my original self,
I become reunited with a deep and eternal person.

■

In the world to come I shall not be asked, "Why were you not Moses?" I
shall be asked, "Why were you not Zusya?"
RABBI ZUSYA

When you are content to be simply yourself and don't compare
or compete, everyone will respect you.
LAO-TZU

BALANCE

a state of equilibrium or parity
characterized by cancellation of all forces
by equal opposing forces

■

I always try to balance the light with the heavy—a few tears of human
spirit in with the sequins and the fringes.
BETTE MIDLER

Just as your car runs more smoothly and requires less energy to go
faster and farther when the wheels are in perfect alignment, you perform better when your thoughts, feelings, emotions, goals, and values
are in balance.
BRIAN TRACY

Believing in our hearts that who we are is enough is the key to a more
satisfying and balanced life.
ELLEN SUE STERN

TWO DECADES AGO, my friend Cynthia Gale learned she had a hopeless form of multiple sclerosis. At the time, she was the youngest person to be a dean at a prestigious college, and her art career was taking off.
Not surprisingly, when doctors' attempts to control her intractable disease
failed, Cynthia felt desperate. "I became legally blind and couldn't use my
hands. I couldn't walk steadily, and I almost died during a clinical trial.
Everything felt out of balance," she said.

Scared that she would never regain control, Cynthia decided to take full
responsibility for rebalancing her life. "I took nothing for granted," she
explained. "I did everything—whether it was eating, cooking, meditating,
cleaning, or feeding my cats—with Zenlike intentionality. Since I could no

longer work, I spent hours just thinking and listening to everything my body was trying to tell me. I asked myself, "How did I get so out of balance? What in my life causes me to stumble? What am I blind to? What centers me?"

Slowly, as she struggled with those questions, Cynthia's disease went into remission, and she saw her life anew. In the year that followed, she left her marriage and began studying art again. She also traveled West, where native healers taught her ceremonies for balancing her inner world with the environment. Today, Cynthia is an acclaimed artist who creates beautiful ceremonial objects dedicated to the healing of our unbalanced planet. She remains symptom free.

According to Elisabeth Kübler-Ross, who pioneered the death and dying movement, "Healing does not necessarily mean to become physically well or to be able to get up and walk around again. Rather, it means achieving a balance between the physical, emotional, intellectual, and spiritual dimensions." For Cynthia, achieving that balance was truly a matter of dying to an old way of life so that she could, indeed, live.

AFFIRMATION

I know that when I take time to listen to my body, mind, and spirit,
I bring more balance into my life.

Where there is sunshine, there is also shade.
KASHMIRI

The best and safest thing is to keep a balance in your life, acknowledge
the great powers around us and in us. If you can do that, and live that
way, you are really a wise man.
EURIPIDES

BEAUTY

*a delightful quality associated with harmony of
form or color: a quality or feature that is most
effective, gratifying, or telling*

■

Think of all the beauty still left around you and be happy.
ANNE FRANK

People are like stained-glass windows. They sparkle and shine when the
sun is out, but when the darkness sets in, their true beauty is revealed
only if there is a light from within.
ELISABETH KÜBLER-ROSS

The pain passes, but the beauty remains.
PIERRE-AUGUSTE RENOIR

WHILE GROWING UP, I never imagined that I could be a beautiful person. One of my earliest memories is of my mother pointing at me while saying, "Other people get blessed with flowers. God gave me an onion."

Although I didn't know exactly what it meant to be a child *and* an onion, I didn't have to be a genius to understand that onions didn't win beauty pageants. My father smelled awful after he ate them raw, and my mother cried as she peeled away the paper-thin skin that served no practical purpose.

If, as Marshall McLuhan said, "the medium is the message," here's how a child who believes she's an onion sees herself: First, I was neither a flower nor beautiful. Second, I smelled bad, and beautiful things smelled good. And third, if I remained thin-skinned, I would be of no purpose to my parents, the world, or myself.

Like all children, I was eager, if not anxious, to please—especially my parents. Afraid that no amount of cleansing would ever stop me from reeking like an onion, and even more fearful that if I scrubbed my thin skin too ambitiously it might all slough off, I chose another tack. I began layering myself with armor that, I hoped, would cover up my offensive qualities and protect my skin. It took many forms. Lots of it encased my feelings and emotions. My wild, unkempt hair sheltered thoughts I needed to keep hidden in my head. And the long-sleeved dark shirts that I wore, even on the hottest summer days, kept the rest of me under wraps.

It wasn't until Arnold Tversky, my high-school English teacher and first mentor, spoke about the joy of peeling away the different layers of an onion to unfold mystery and understand complexity that I began intimating there might be more to me than what met my mother's eye. "Given enough time to grow, even onions sprout beautiful flowers," Arnold said to me. "And you know where all that beauty comes from? Their core."

■

AFFIRMATION

The beauty I see in the world is a reflection of the beauty hidden inside me.

■

A beautiful thing is never perfect.
EGYPTIAN PROVERB

He hath made every thing beautiful in his time.
ECCLESIASTES

BELIEF

*mental acceptance and conviction of the truth,
actuality, or validity of something*

■

If you believe you can, you probably can.
If you believe you won't, you most assuredly won't.
Belief is the ignition switch that gets you off the launching pad.
DENNIS WAITLEY

Before the art of medicine comes the art of belief.
DEEPAK CHOPRA

Learned helplessness is the giving-up reaction,
the quitting response that follows from the
belief that whatever you do doesn't matter.
MARTIN SELIGMAN

UPON LEARNING THAT I might have a life-threatening illness, my mind begin racing in all directions as I began to absorb the body-shocking news and inventory my belief system. Do I believe my doctor? Do I believe *in* my doctor? What do I believe about traditional medicine? What do I believe about complementary medicine? What do I believe about the outcome of this disease? What do others who have it believe?

Rachel Naomi Remen, M.D., knows a lot about beliefs, both her own and others'. She is an acclaimed author, cofounder and medical director of the Commonweal Cancer Help Program in Bolinas, California, and a wounded healer who has lived with a life-threatening illness for over four decades. During an interview with PBS journalist Bill Moyers, she discussed the relationship between the healing process and beliefs:

You weren't born with your beliefs. Some of your beliefs may help you to live, and some of them may not. And you need to be able to sort them out, because only the ones that are true, only the ones that can help you to live, are the ones you want to keep. Let me give you an image. I bought a little, falling-down cabin on the top of a mountain. It was so bad that a friend said, Oh Rachel, you bought this? But with two carpenters, an electrician, and a plumber, we have remodeled the whole thing in three years.

We started by just throwing things away—bathtubs, light fixtures, windows. I kept hearing my father's voice saying, "That's a perfectly good light fixture, why are you throwing it away?" We kept throwing away more and more things, and with everything we threw away, the building became more whole. It had more integrity. Finally, we had thrown away everything that didn't belong. You know, we may think we need to be more in order to be whole. But in some ways, we need to be less. We need to let go, to throw away everything that isn't us in order to be more whole. . . . You want to live as long as you can, but don't you want to live well?

■

AFFIRMATION

When I discard beliefs that don't serve me, I become more whole.

■

To believe with certainty, we must begin by doubting.
POLISH PROVERB

All things can be done for the one who believes.
MARK 9:23

BLESSING

something promoting or contributing to happiness, well-being, or prosperity; a boon

■

May the force be with you.
GEORGE LUCAS

This is the wisdom: If we bless our bodies, they will bless us.
GLORIA STEINEM

Health . . . is the first and greatest of all blessings.
LORD CHESTERFIELD

L AST WINTER, I visited Verne Edwards for the first time in more than twenty-five years. Although occasional letters, cards, phone calls, and e-mail helped me to stay in touch with my college mentor, whenever we planned to meet, random acts of life and weather canceled them. And so time passed, and for a quarter of a century the slightly-built man who sported a touch of curmudgeon and I lived in our own worlds only two hours apart.

But the winter of 2000 was different. For me it was a cold, icy time when the pain and discontent I felt over my brush with a life-threatening illness kept cutting into me like the blade of my surgeon's knife. And yet it was also a winter where I felt ablaze with love, support, and gifts of self-healing that I had never experienced before. In gratitude for the life I saw ahead of me, I wanted to look back at my past and knew I needed to see Verne.

When we met again, I instantly recognized my dapper, snowy-haired journalism professor. Turning toward me, he did a double take. Over lunch, as our conversation drifted into the past, I began thanking him for his blessings—for telling me that I had what it took to become a successful writer; for being a tough but fair taskmaster; for believing in me when I didn't; for bailing a renegade out of all kinds of deep, smelly stuff; for listening; for taking the risk to stand up to those whose self-serving interests might have harmed me; and for being so trustworthy and trusting. In turn, his eyes, expressions, and words thanked me.

When, I wonder, does a blessing become a blessing? Is it when it's thought of? When it's spoken? When it's heard, or when it's acknowledged—not just in the head but in the heart? In his poem "Vacillation," William Butler Yeats wrote that, sometime after his fiftieth birthday, he was sitting alone in a coffee shop and knew "of a sudden" that he was "blessed and could bless." When Verne and I embraced and then parted on that winter day in Delaware, Ohio, I knew that I was blessed and had blessed.

■

■

A wise man should consider that health
is the greatest of human blessings.
HIPPOCRATES

When difficulties are overcome, they begin blessing.
PROVERB

BODY

*the entire material or
physical structure of an organism*

■

It's also helpful to realize that this very body that we have, that's
sitting right here, right now . . . with its aches and its pleasures . . . is
exactly what we need to be fully human, fully awake, fully alive.
PEMA CHÖDRÖN

When the body is finally listened to . . . it becomes eloquent. It's like
changing a fiddle into a Stradivarius. It gets much more highly attuned.
MARION WOODMAN

My body taught me many things, all of them filled with soul: how to dance
and make love, mourn and make music; now it is teaching me how to heal. I
am learning to heed the shifting currents of my body—the subtle changes
in temperature, muscle tension, thought and mood—the way a sailor rides
the wind by reading the ripples on the water.
KAT DUFF

THE LEGENDARY DANCER Martha Graham once wrote, "You will know
the wonders of the human body because there is nothing more wonderful. The next time you look into the mirror, just look at the way the ears
rest next to the head; look at the way the hairline grows; think of all the little bones in your wrist. It is a miracle."

A miracle indeed. After my children were born, I counted and kissed all their
fingers and toes. I also spent time gently cleaning debris from their nostrils,
ears, genitals, eyes, and skin folds and never imagined that there were parts of
their bodies that should be avoided or ignored. When I bathed them, one hand
would cradle their wobbly necks and soft heads while the other would pour
water over their heads or massage their tiny limbs. Then I'd lovingly pat them

dry and rub soothing oils on their backs and sensitive bottoms. Such care. In those nurturing moments, I repeatedly helped to heal the trauma their bodies had experienced upon leaving the safety of my womb. However, it wasn't until years later that I realized how much I had ignored my own body and how it, too, yearned for my healing touch.

Novalis said, "There is only *one* temple in the world and that is the human body." Now ask yourself:

- When was the last time I looked at my body and felt each part was a miracle?
- When was the last time I thanked these parts for doing their jobs so seamlessly?
- What might I do differently to help harmonize parts that do not feel well?
- How might I thank these parts for being my steadiest companions all these years? With words? By my deeds?

■

AFFIRMATION

I thank all the different parts of my body for
dancing with each other all these years.

■

Is not the body the soul's house? Then why should we
not take care of the house that it fall not into ruins?
PHILO

The human body is vapor materialized by
sunshine mixed with the life of the stars.
PARACELSUS

BREATH

the air inhaled and exhaled in respiration;

spirit or vitality

■

Our breathing is the fragile vessel
that carries us from birth to death.
FREDERICK LEBOYER

Breath opens us up. It fills every space that is empty.
DEBORAH MORRIS CORYELL

Breathe on me, breath of God,
fill me with life anew,
that I may love what thou dost love,
and do what thou wouldst do.
EDWIN HATCH

THROUGHOUT MY LIFE, I have been privileged to be with several people when they drew their last breath. Only once was I with someone
who couldn't draw his first. That person was my son, Evan.

My pregnancy went smoothly for eight months until a bacterial infection
caused me to be bedridden with high fever, chills, and nausea. Although my
obstetrician reassured me that my baby would be fine, I harbored doubts.
No longer did this gestating life vigorously kick my abdomen and move
around. All I felt was an occasional flutter. Some days I felt nothing at all.

On October 26, 1971, I started having contractions. Past experience
with the birth of my daughter suggested I get to the hospital immediately.
By the time I arrived in the emergency room, the baby was well on its way,
and I had no choice but to deliver it naturally.

"Breathe. Breathe. Breathe like this," the nurse kept instructing me between orders to push and pant and pant and stop pushing. "Breathing will ease the pain. Breathing will help your baby. Just breathe. For crying out loud, breathe!" I wanted to, and tried to, but thieves named fear and confusion kept stealing my breath over and over again, until finally after one huge push I heard the words, "It's a boy." But before I could sigh with relief, I was again robbed of my breath. Why wasn't my baby crying? Why was he limp? Why were people rushing everywhere? I tried shouting, "What's happening?" but my breathless voice couldn't push the words out. "Your son's just having a small problem," said a nurse. Small problem, indeed. My baby wasn't breathing—he was not yet alive.

Within moments the doctor aspirated thick mucous blocking Evan's tiny air passages. In response, my new son inhaled a deep breath that flooded his skin with color and exhaled a loud cry announcing, "I am!" And when, at last, they placed this living soul in my arms, instead of first counting his fingers and toes, I just listened to the healing sounds of us breathing in and breathing out, breathing in and breathing out . . .

■

AFFIRMATION

With every breath, I fill myself with life anew.

■

**With every inhalation I create the universe,
with every exhalation I destroy it.**
ZEN PROVERB

**There is one way of breathing that is shameful and constricted.
Then there's another way, a breath of love
that takes you all the way to infinity.**
JALAL-UDDIN RUMI

[23]

CHALLENGE

*a test of one's abilities or resources in a
demanding but stimulating undertaking*

■

The challenge is to turn midnight into days, pain into power.
If you're swimming, and there's a stiff wind and a vicious storm
coming, you can't stop swimming and explain the storm away.
You've got to keep kicking.
JESSE JACKSON

There is a tide in the affairs of men which
taken at the flood leads on to fortune.
WILLIAM SHAKESPEARE

Life's challenges are not supposed to paralyze you,
they're supposed to help you discover who you are.
BERNICE JOHNSON REAGON

WHETHER IT'S CHOOSING to climb a mountain or to climb into a bed
for dialysis or to climb over the ruins of some part of our lives, once
we accept a challenge, we step into the world of the unknown and it forever
changes us. Moreover, I would guess that, once on the other side of the most
serious challenges that we've accepted, most of us have felt strengthened by
the experience.

In a few days, a dear friend will enter a month-long alcohol abuse rehabilitation program. The challenges he faces for the sake of this healing journey are enormous. Along the way he will be challenged to give up living life
as an alcoholic or else risk being given up by his family, friends, and business associates. He will have to give up some of his pride and the tempta-
tion to place blame for his woes outside himself. I imagine the false truths

that supported his justification for using alcohol and then abusing it will be sacrificed. He must also be prepared to be challenged by new truths that will open old wounds and turn his familiar world upside down.

When faced with accepting or rejecting serious ventures that challenge the whole of our personalities, psychologist Carl G. Jung says that caution has its place but we cannot refuse our support. "If we oppose it, we are trying to suppress what is best in man—his daring and his aspirations. And should we succeed, we should only have stood in the way of that invaluable experience which might have given a meaning to life. What would have happened if Paul had allowed himself to be talked out of his journey to Damascus?"

In meeting a challenge, we become witnesses to our ability to go where we haven't gone before, do what we've never done before, and arrive at a new place in our lives. Indeed, once witnessed, the courage, fortitude, self-trust, and even the humility that helped carry us through can never be "unwitnessed."

■

AFFIRMATION

That which challenges me most strengthens me.

■

Difficulties strengthen the mind, as labor does the body.
SENECA

When difficulties are overcome, they begin blessing.
PROVERB

CHANGE

*to cause to be different; to give a completely dif-
ferent form or appearance to; to transform*

■

The first step toward change is acceptance. Once you accept
yourself, you open the door to change. That's all you have to do.
Change is not something you do, it's something you allow.
WIL GARCIA

We cannot change anything unless we accept it.
Condemnation does not liberate, it oppresses.
CARL JUNG

The need for change bulldozed a road down the center of my mind.
MAYA ANGELOU

"GOD, GRANT ME the serenity to accept the things I cannot change, the courage to change the things I can, and the wisdom to know the difference." Throughout the world, people who abuse addictive substances religiously recite theologian Reinhold Niebuhr's words. In the turbulent sea of change that accompanies their desire to no longer be sucked into self-destructive and abusive behaviors, these reassuring words about acceptance, courage, and wisdom anchor them.

Why, I wonder during times of transition, do I feel so anxious and shaky? "What in me resists accepting the fact that there are things I cannot change?" I ask. "Where will I find the courage to change the things I can? And what about this thing called wisdom that helps me differentiate between my positive and negative responses to changes in my life? Do I have what it takes to really *know* the difference?"

As people worldwide—rich, poor, educated, illiterate, young, elderly, Republican, Democratic, Independent, religious, agnostic, atheistic—gather daily at Alcoholics Anonymous and many other mutual support group meetings, they become living legacies who demonstrate humanity's inherent desire to make changes for life-enhancing, healing reasons. Indeed, as these courageous people stand before their peers to speak truthfully about their devastating and destructive lives, they publicly confess that what they stand for is change. And, in the process, the greatest lesson their self-disclosure may teach others is not that they are embracing change just because they want *their* lives to be different, but because they also want to make a difference to those whom they love, their community, and the world.

■

AFFIRMATION

May it not bother me to find that I am ever-changing
and not the same person from day to day.

■

If you realize that all things change,
there is nothing you will try to hold onto.
TAO TE CHING

Would that life were like the shadow cast by a wall or a tree,
but it is like the shadow of a bird in flight.
TALMUD

CHAOS

*a condition or place of
great disorder or confusion*

■

You need chaos in your soul to give birth to a dancing star.
FRIEDRICH NIETZSCHE

Where do we come from? Where are we going? That is what every
heart is shouting, what every head is asking as it beats on chaos.
NIKOS KAZANTZAKIS

Chaos often breeds life, when order breeds habit.
HENRY BROOKS ADAMS

IN THE BEGINNING, creation myths spontaneously arose worldwide. In
many of these stories, the opening sentences describe a chaotic state of
nonbeing. Then, through supernatural intervention, nothingness is transformed into a harmonious and balanced world. Here are the ways in which
some of these myths describe the chaos:

GREEK: In the beginning was Chaos and darkness. Chaos was a great vast sea
in which all the elements were mixed together without form.
GERMANIC: In the beginning was the great void, Ginnungagap. A fiery
region developed to the south and a windy, icy region to the north.
Together they produced chaos and out of chaos sprang life.
CHINESE: In the beginning was a huge black egg containing chaos and a
mixture of yin-yang.
JAPANESE: In the beginning there was nothing but a vast oily sea of Chaos that
contained a mix of all the elements.

[28]

HUNGARIAN:
  The seeds of the Holy Sea break out of your shell.
  The eternal sea's waves are waving, and rolling.
  Their waves are rocking and their foam is hissing.
  There is no earth yet anywhere . . .
JUDEO-CHRISTIAN: In the beginning God created the heaven and the earth.
  And the earth was without form, and void; and darkness was upon the face
  of the deep. . . . And God saw all that He had made, and found it very good.

Physical, emotional, and spiritual illnesses can hurl us into the void these myths describe. Feeling frightened and untethered, we may frantically wonder whether or not we can survive the ravages of the stormy, oily, hissing sea of despair, confusion, and loneliness around us. However, if we take seriously what these timeless stories do, we learn that our potential to create calm and healing may rest within the eye of the storm that is causing our angst. Indeed, when we choose to create a worldview that supports our greater good and well-being, we, too, discover that out of chaos comes new life—new life that is "very good."

■

AFFIRMATION

When I create new life out of my darkness,
I bring to light something "very good."

■

In the beginning, the world was nothing but a quagmire.
AINU

Skillful pilots gain their reputation from storms and tempests.
EPICTETUS

CHOICE

*the act of choosing; selection; the power, right,
or liberty to choose; option*

■

When a defining moment comes along, you can do one of two things.
Define the moment, or let the moment define you.
TIN CUP

Before my accident, there were ten thousand things I could do.
I could spend the rest of my life dwelling on the things that I had lost,
but instead I chose to focus on the nine thousand I still had left.
W. MITCHELL

One cannot get through life without pain. . . .
What we can do is choose how to use the pain life presents to us.
BERNIE SIEGEL

ONE DAY, MY mother asked, "Do you want to take ballet or music lessons? It's your choice." I was five years old and didn't know. So I went outside to sit on our stoop and think. Later, my mother came out and found me sobbing. "Why are you crying?" she asked. "Because it's really hard to make a choice," I wailed.

Almost five decades later, I still wail over hard choices. Sometimes I feel like I've been stoop-sitting for days, weeks, or even years before both my heart and mind agree on a decision. I know it felt that way when after two years of saying "Should I or shouldn't I?" I suddenly woke up one day and knew I had to ask my first husband for a divorce.

I also spent time stoop-sitting when my surgeon told me to choose between having a mastectomy without further treatment or a lumpectomy and thirty-three radiation treatments. For days I struggled in the tension of painful opposites: "To keep or not to keep my left breast? What a #$%*&!@!%¢§#% choice."

Just months after my lumpectomy, my mother lay in a Florida hospital attached to life support equipment. A doctor's defiant decision to put her on a respirator defiled her living will. I wanted the tube removed so she could die as she wished—peacefully and with dignity. However, my mother's rabbi, her authority on the Jewish law that she dearly loved, said, "No. Now God must decide what to do."

"But the Jewish Kabbalah says, 'Man was created for the sake of choice,' " said the voice inside my head.

Throughout the night, I sobbed as ambiguity pulled me from one side of the stoop to the other: "What's the cost and promise of removing life support? What's the cost and promise of *not* removing it? What should I do?" The next morning, I entered the hospital tallying the pros and cons and finally knew.

■

AFFIRMATION

I am responsible for my own well-being.
My choices influence the quality of my days.

■

No choice is also a choice.
YIDDISH PROVERB

It is your own convictions which compel you,
that is, choice compels choice.
EPICTETUS

COMFORT

to soothe in time of affliction or distress;
to ease physically; relieve

■

Clasp my hand, dear friend, I am dying.
CONTE VITTORIO ALFIERI (AS HE WAS DYING)

Comfort the afflicted and afflict the comfortable.
FINLEY PETER DUNNE

When you have nothing left but God,
you become aware that God is enough.
GUIDEPOSTS

SHORTLY AFTER BERNADIN Hospice House in Columbia, South Carolina, opened its doors in April 2000, a young feral cat showing up whenever patients sat outside. According to my friend Libby Green, marketing director of this facility for those with life-limiting illnesses, the patients love feeding and stroking the little black-and-white feline they named Whiskers. One day, the staff found her inside on the bed of a three-year-old girl who was dying of leukemia. Although patients can keep domestic pets at this hospice, no one knew Whiskers's health history. So a nurse put her out. But, said Libby, no matter how many times the staff removed her, Whiskers would sneak back in to nestle alongside that child. The day after the little girl died, she added, Whiskers began visiting other patients.

When a local vet heard about Whiskers, he voluntarily spayed and inoculated her so she could roam freely. Since then, Whiskers has arrived daily in time to accompany the nurses on their morning rounds. Once finished, she then returns to the room of whichever patient is closest to death. "We don't know how Whiskers knows," says Libby, "she just does. It's so uncanny, but if we have two patients dying at the same time, Whiskers splits her time between them."

Not too long ago, an elderly patient at Bernardin who was near death suddenly opened her eyes. "Shhh!," she said. "He's here." Then, according to Libby, "she began staring at something invisible to others in the room. At that moment, Whiskers came in and immediately froze and focused on the same invisible object as the patient. Whiskers didn't move until the woman closed her eyes."

Although the staff jokes that Whiskers is the reincarnation of the first patient who died at Bernadin, they take seriously their belief that she's a gift from God sent to comfort their patients. Unlike the biblical character Job, whose visitors' attempts to console him drove him deeper and deeper into despair and darkness, Whiskers's visits brighten and comfort the dying as they face their darkest hour.

■

AFFIRMATION

More and more I am grateful for that which comforts me.

■

Yea, though I walk through the valley of the shadow of death,
I will fear no evil; for thou art with me;
thy rod and thy staff they comfort me.
PSALMS 23:4

My bed shall comfort me, my couch shall ease my complaint.
JOB 7:13

COMMITMENT

the state of being bound emotionally or intellectually to a course of action or to another person or persons; a pledge to do

■

Resolve that whatever you do, you will bring the whole man to it;
that you will fling the whole weight of your being into it.
ORISON SWETT MARDEN

You need to make a commitment, and once you make it,
then life will give you some answers.
LES BROWN

Unless commitment is made,
there are only promises and hopes, but no plans.
PETER F. DRUCKER

EVER SINCE HE got an e-mail from his sister saying that a distant cousin needed a lung transplant, Steve Miceli, thirty-three, has been living the question, "Should I give him one of mine?"

"Tell me about your cousin," I said after hearing about my friend Steve's struggle to determine whether or not to donate one of the five lobes that made up his lungs.

"He's fifty," said Steve, "and I believe he's also the oldest living cystic fibrosis patient in the world. His lungs are failing and a transplant is his only hope. He doesn't need just one lung. He needs two, which means two donors. All I know right now is that our blood types match."

"You must really love him," I replied.

"No, I just met him once—last summer. We only talked for a few minutes. It wasn't like we got to know each other."

According to Steve, his immediate response to the e-mail was to give his cousin his lung. "It sounds so simplistic, but I felt the way you feel when you drive by someone you know at a bus stop and ask if they need a ride. Of course, I could do this. But when I really stopped to think, I knew it would be a difficult decision. Whatever I choose to do also affects my wife and daughters."

For the next two hours, Steve talked about the discernment process to which he had committed himself. He was gathering information about transplants and contacting medical centers where they were performed. He planned to talk to organ donors and recipients. He was trying to determine the cost and promise of donating his lung and the cost and promise of not doing it. He was mining his psyche and soul to see if he could dig up repressed feelings. If he didn't donate his lung, he wondered, could he make another gift—gifts of blood or patient advocacy, perhaps?

"I am committed to staying with this process—wherever it leads me," he said as we left. "And you know what? Maybe it's the process, not the outcome, that this is all about."

■

AFFIRMATION

My healing journey begins with my commitment to the healing process.

■

Little by little the bird builds its nest.
FRENCH PROVERB

Therefore diligently observe the words of this covenant, in order that
you may succeed in everything that you do.
DEUTERONOMY 29:9

[35]

COMMUNITY

a unified body of individuals.

■

No man is an island, entire of itself;
every man is a piece of the continent.
JOHN DONNE

I am part of all that I have met.
ALFRED, LORD TENNYSON

They keep intact the close chain of sympathetic responses in which
man first securely established himself as irrevocably human:
these friendly eyes are the indispensable mirror
in which the self beholds its own image.
LEWIS MUMFORD

IN THE LATE 1990s, psychiatrist David Spiegel published a study showing that women with metastatic breast cancer who belonged to a support
group lived longer. Although I'm a real introvert who considers more than
two people in a room a crowd, those findings didn't surprise me. Even I
admit to occasionally feeling strong urges to connect with like-minded
friends, peers, and my faith community just for the health of it. In fact, I
have no doubt that our universal, innate yearning to be in relationship with
others is, in part, rooted in a deep, abiding truth that healthy communities
offer us protective immunity.

During times of illness and grievous personal loss, communities of
friends, relatives, and even strangers gather round to nourish and fortify us
physically, spiritually and emotionally by helping us to endure our pain, heal
our wounds, and continue to say "Yes!" to life. Without asking, they eagerly
pray for our health and survival, not just with words, but with deeds, too.
They show up at our doorsteps and hospital beds with casseroles, cakes,

cards, and other tokens of their concern. They give us a hero's "Hurrah" for making strides we may consider insignificant. They magically appear to pick up the balls we drop and keep them in play. And, at those times when the fact that we have nothing to say says it all, they just sit in silence with us.

It's no surprise to me that Spiegel's study showed that we do far better when we connect with one another. After my treatments for breast cancer ended, I started a support group. At the first meeting, each woman talked about her hopes, fears, and concerns about the future. While watching heads nod in agreement, I felt my own head doing the same. Looking into the eyes of those around me, I saw that I didn't have to experience exactly what each woman went through to know her story was my story. We were, that night and forever more, all in this together.

■

AFFIRMATION

I surround myself with love, caring, support, and strength
when I invite assistance from friends, loved ones, and even strangers.

■

Visitors' footfalls are like medicine; they heal the sick.
BANTU PROVERB

Company in distress makes trouble less.
FRENCH PROVERB

COMPASSION

deep awareness of the suffering of another cou-
pled with the wish to relieve it

∎

There is nothing heavier than compassion. Not even one's own pain
weighs so heavy as the pain one feels with someone, for someone, a pain
intensified by the imagination and prolonged by a hundred echoes.

MILAN KUNDERA

Compassion is bringing our deepest truth into our actions, no matter
how much the world seems to resist, because that is ultimately what we
have to give this world and one another.

RAM DASS

It is the experience of touching the pain of others that is the key to
change.... Compassion is a sign of transformation.

JIM WALLIS

As MY MOTHER lay dying of heart failure, her Orthodox rabbi came to
visit her in the hospital. Anxiously, I extended my hand to shake his—
momentarily forgetting that Jewish law forbade him to touch women. Upon
realizing my mistake, I apologized. "It's not necessary," he said. "There are
greater concerns right now."

He then went to the foot of my mother's bed and stood shaking his head.
Against the wishes of my mother's living will, hospital personnel had inserted a ventilator tube into her chest. It grotesquely distorted her tiny, pale
face. Eighteen other wires and tubes were attached to her body. We all
found it hard to believe that the unconscious person lying there was Muriel.
"She was doing so well. What happened?" her rabbi asked. "I can't believe it."

Their relationship was special. Years earlier, when my mother rediscovered her Jewish roots, this knowledgeable man, half her age, became her trustworthy mentor. Weekly, the small, black-bearded and black-suited rabbi and the woman with a blonde pageboy haircut, who wore boldly colored caftans, would meet to discuss all aspects of Judaism—especially the laws governing daily life. On special occasions, the rabbi invited Mom to share a meal with his wife and five small children. Despite the fact that he couldn't hug his favorite student, she always felt warmly embraced by his love.

Now that relationship, as each knew it, was ending. Moving closer to her bedside, the rabbi began reciting prayers in Hebrew. Rhythmically, he swayed as his soothing, singsong voice became a counterpoint to the menacing, mechanical sounds the monitors made. Finally, the rabbi closed his prayer book and again stood sorrowfully beside my mother. Then, reaching out, he clasped her hand in his.

■

AFFIRMATION

Compassion that comes from the heart knows no bounds.

■

He, our Father, He hath shown His mercy unto me.
In peace I walk the straight road.
CHEYENNE PROVERB

But a certain Samaritan, as he journeyed, came where he was: and
when he saw him, he had compassion on him.
And went to him, and bound up his wounds . . . and took care of him.
LUKE 10:33-35

CONFESS

*to disclose (something damaging or
inconvenient to oneself); admit*

■

It is the confession, not the priest, that gives us absolution.
OSCAR WILDE

A confession has to be part of your new life.
LUDWIG WITTGENSTEIN

Men will confess to treason, murder, arson, false teeth or a wig. How
many of them will own up to a lack of humor?
FRANK MOORE COLBY

THEY SAY THAT confessing is good for the soul. I'd go a step further and
say that confessing our truth is healing, and it's healing not just for our
souls, but for our bodies and emotions, too. Take Zachary's confession, for
example.

A few years ago, this gentle, slightly stooped, mentally challenged man
began attending Ted's early Sunday service. Usually, only fifteen to twenty
regular worshippers show up, and they sit close together in the choir loft in
front of the altar. Zachary would always arrive late and look as though he had
slept in his clothes. A ten-gallon cowboy hat usually topped his small frame,
and a big metal medallion from a Cadillac always hung on a chain around his
neck. Because he never followed the liturgy, no one knew if Zachary was lit-
erate. He would just sit quietly throughout the service, or else he would follow everyone else's lead and stand, sit, and receive blessings when they did.
The only time Zachary interacted with the other worshippers was when
everyone exchanged handshakes and said "Peace be with you."

One Sunday, the readings were about the Ten Commandments. As Ted began delivering his sermon, Zachary, as usual, wandered in late. Ted paused, smiled, invited him to sit down, and then started over again. Zachary listened intently for a few minutes, but then, in a loud, monotone voice, interrupted. "Father," he said in front of everyone, "Father, am I forgiven? Am I forgiven, Father, because I've broken all but one of the commandments?"

Ted didn't ask Zachary about the lone commandment that wasn't broken, and he didn't ask him about the nine that were. He did assure Zachary that God forgave him, and when he did, Zachary stood straight up, smiled, and with tears said, "Thank you, Father. I've never told anyone that. But today I told you. Thank you, Father, thank you. I feel so different inside."

Later, at the main Sunday service, Ted ditched his prepared sermon and walked out into the aisle to tell the congregation about Zachary. He talked about Zachary's question, about his smile, about his tears, and about how our willingness to acknowledge we've missed the mark helps to relieve us of our burdens and to stand up straight.

■

AFFIRMATION

My confessions help to straighten and heal the bent parts of me.

■

Open confession is good for the soul.
SCOTTISH PROVERB

A sin confessed is half forgiven.
FRENCH PROVERB

COURAGE

*the state or quality of mind or spirit that
enables one to face danger, fear, or vicissitudes
with self-possession, confidence, and resolution*

■

Life shrinks or expands in proportion to one's courage.
ANAÏS NIN

Not everything that is faced can be changed,
but nothing can be changed until it is faced.
JAMES BALDWIN

We learn to fly not by becoming fearless,
but by the daily practice of courage.
SAM KEEN

IN 1988, I went on a rugged Outward Bound sailing expedition for adults off the coast of Maine. The famed Outward Bound courses are designed to be physically, mentally, and emotionally demanding experiential learning adventures. Many people claim Outward Bound changed their lives. I'm one of them.

On Outward Bound, I attempted things I had never done before. I plunged into a 47° ocean. I lived with twelve other adults on a boat that had no galley or head. I slept sardine style on top of oars. I rock-climbed to overcome a fear of heights only a klutz can have. I lived solo on an uninhabited island for two and a half days, and I did a high ropes course that is so challenging it's used to train soldiers. By the time my expedition ended, Outward Bound had taught me plenty about facing my fears, but not as much as my shipmate Gerald did.

Gerald, a Roman Catholic priest in his fifties, approached most exercises as we all did—with some trepidation countered by an overriding determination to get on with it. That is, until we got to the infamous ropes course—a series of graduated challenges strung amongst trees overlooking a high, rocky cliff. On the second level, Gerald froze. Faced with having to make a small leap in mid air to get from his log to another, he became paralyzed. After all our attempts to encourage him failed, one of the leaders asked Gerald one simple question. "What's stopping you?" she shouted up. "I don't know. I don't know," he wailed back. "Would you like me to help you?" she asked. "No," he barked angrily. "I'm just stupid Mr. Bumbles, stupid Mr. Bumbles."

"Gerald!" she said. "When was the last time someone called you that?" Shocked, he sat down on the log to think. "I was twelve," he answered softly. Then, before we could wonder what would follow, Gerald grabbed a support rope, hoisted himself up, set his sights on the other log, leapt across the tiny chasm, and just kept on going—higher and higher toward the top.

■

AFFIRMATION

Day by day I am learning to fly, not by becoming fearless,
but through the practice of courage.

■

Wealth lost—something lost; Honor lost—much lost;
Courage lost—all lost.
GERMAN PROVERB

If you are afraid of something, you give it power over you.
MOROCCAN PROVERB

CREATIVITY

*having the ability or power to create; character-
ized by originality and expressiveness*

■

There are only four colors, ten digits, and seven notes;
it's what we do with them that's important.
RUTH ROSS

Uncertainty and mystery are energies of life. Don't let them scare you
unduly, for they keep boredom at bay and spark creativity.
R.I. FITZHENRY

Creativity puts order into chaos, life into the inert,
and beauty into the ordinary.
EDWARD J. LAVIN

THERE'S A CREATOR that resides inside of each of us who yearns to guide us to a healing path. Whenever he or she calls to us from our imagination, we can be assured it's to give us a glimpse of what life outside the box might be about—life that can be more colorful, viewed through a different lens, filled with texture, and in touch with untapped healing energies lying dormant in our bodies, psyches, and souls.

My friend Sandra Ingerman, author of *Medicine for the Earth* and *Soul Retrieval*, is a psychotherapist who incorporates ancient healing rituals into her workshops and private practice. "In working with people who are facing life-threatening illnesses, I notice a significant pattern," she says. "People who come to me for a one-time 'fix' and refuse to look at making changes in their lives get better for a time, but might eventually fall ill again." By contrast, she has found that clients who decide to use their creative energy to help themselves express life-supportive changes have a greater tendency to beat the odds and live good lives. "Even if they cannot be cured, their desire to be creators who shape and color the life they are living ensures healing."

Sandy believes that everyone bears the responsibility of choosing how to create health in his or her life and then maintain it. The first key to opening up a palette of possibilities is to make a conscious decision to bring into being a healthy present and future, she says. Next comes trusting that you have both the innate ability and the right to use your creative energy in any way that's satisfying for you. And the final key is to find the courage to take action and not let the judgments of others—living or dead—stifle the creativity that's your birthright.

"In my work," says Sandy, "I teach that the word *power* means the ability to use energy and transform it. Whenever we talk about healing, we are really talking about taking responsibility for creatively transforming our energy—about crafting it into life-supportive and positive futures and thereby becoming power-filled."

AFFIRMATION

I possess the power I need to create the life I want to live.

Every art requires the whole person.
FRENCH PROVERB

The End of every maker is himself.
SAINT THOMAS AQUINAS

DANCE

*to move rhythmically, usually to music, using
prescribed or improvised steps and gestures*

■

Life is movement, movement is life.
To live is to move, to move is to be alive.
MIRKA KNASTER

We should consider every day lost in which we
have not danced at least once.
FRIEDRICH NIETZSCHE

It's the heart afraid of breaking that never learns to dance.
AMANDA MCBROOM

LIKE LOTS OF young girls, Mary Verdi-Fletcher always dreamed of
becoming a dancer. From childhood on, she says, something in her body,
psyche, and soul kept urging her to use dance to know time, space, and her
place in the world in a new way. So against all odds, Mary, who has spina
bifida and uses a wheelchair instead of her legs for mobility, chose to dance
her way through life.

I met Mary fifteen years ago when she rolled up to meet me in a restau-
rant for the first of many interviews I would have with her. She told me then
that her vision was not only to dance, but to help others discover that, even
if they couldn't leap, dancing would let their souls soar. Today, Dancing
Wheels, Mary's internationally acclaimed troupe of professional dancers
with and without disabilities, performs at over 150 educational
lecture/demonstrations and formal dance concerts annually. "It doesn't matter where I'm dancing—whether it's before a group of elementary school
students or six thousand people at a benefit hosted by actor Christopher

Reeve—I always feel as though the dance dances me. I merely become a vessel for something that allows me to transcend my body and my disability."

Several years ago, when Mary's kidneys failed her, she came to know her body, mind, spirit, and the healing power of dance more intimately. While awaiting an organ transplant from her husband, she lived on dialysis—without her kidneys—for four months. Yet she danced in her studio and before audiences the entire time. "It became so clear to me that dancing was more about my spirit than my body. It's what healed me. Dancing allowed me to get beyond my pains, aches, limitations, and fears, and I believe it can do that for each one of us. Wholeness isn't about limbs. When you move any parts of your body to music, you open pathways in your heart that help you to express all kinds of emotions—joy, pleasure, anger, rage, sadness, happiness. This helps you discover things about yourself that you might not have known before. When that happens, your self-image changes, and ultimately you experience more of life and what it means to be alive."

■

AFFIRMATION

When I dance with life, my soul begins to soar.

■

If you can walk you can dance. If you can talk you can sing.
ZIMBABWE PROVERB

Whatever is flexible and flowing will tend to grow. Whatever is rigid
and blocked will wither and die.
TAO TE CHING

DARKNESS

lacking or having very little light

■

In a dark time the eye begins to see.
THEODORE ROETHKE

When it gets dark enough, you can see the stars.
LEE SALK

I can see, and that is why I can be happy, in what you call the dark, but
which to me is golden. I can see a God-made world,
not a man-made world.
HELEN KELLER

IN THE PARABLE of the prodigal son, a young man asks his father for his
inheritance and takes off to go to a far country. We're not told why he
feels compelled to leave, just that once he's away, he squanders away all his
resources. He must then work as a pig herder—a lowly, disgusting job—in
order to survive. Suddenly, in the midst of literally wallowing in the utmost
darkness, we learn that the prodigal son "comes to himself" and immediately returns home. As he approaches his house, his father warmly greets
and embraces him.

Whenever we suffer from a serious illness or loss, we, too, may feel
exiled to a far country that seems dark and frightening. The signposts in this
country don't help. Instead of guiding us out, it may seem that they only
point to places in our bodies, minds, and spirits that lead us even deeper
into the void. Anxiously, we may begin to look for any opportunity to flee
and return to a world that, while not ideal, felt certain and secure.

Sometimes, through denial, medication, mind-altering substances, and
keeping busy, we do feel like we've temporarily escaped from this strange
and unfriendly place. But without those crutches, we need only to look

around us to know that the only way out of the darkness is to go through it and risk encounters with the scary creatures of the night that dwell there.

In the end, the prodigal son became the hero of his own story, and a grand party was held in his honor. For us to be the heroes and heroines of ours, we must leave what's familiar and confront repressed and painful truths. Each has been waiting a long time for us to face them. Each awaits the opportunity to share something we must know in order to move through the darkness and into a healing light. Only then can we "come to ourselves" and truly celebrate the healing that homecoming brings.

■

AFFIRMATION

Each step through the darkness leads to a healing light.

■

Better to light one small candle than to curse the darkness.
CHINESE PROVERB

Darkness within darkness—the gateway to all understanding.
LAO-TZU

DOUBT

to be undecided or skeptical about

■

When we are not sure, we are alive.
GRAHAM GREENE

Faith and doubt both are needed, but not as antagonists, but working
side by side to take us around the unknown curve.
LILLIAN SMITH

When nothing is sure, everything is possible.
MARGARET DRABBLE

ERIC SEVAREID, THE television news commentator, once said that his self-imposed rule was to retain the courage of his doubts as well as his convictions, "in this world of dangerously passionate certainties."

On the day my surgeon told me I could have either a mastectomy that would remove my left breast with no additional treatment or a lumpectomy followed by radiation, I was convinced I would choose the former. "Why subject myself to radiation? The last time I wore a low-cut dress was to my senior prom. Ted loves *me*," I reasoned.

Although I said nothing, my physician sensed I favored the mastectomy. "Nothing about your condition indicates you should do something radical," he advised. "Take a few days to think about it."

Convinced that I knew which way I'd go, I was surprised to find doubts surfacing before I left the examining room. "Where are they coming from and why?" I wondered. "What might they be trying to tell me?"

Over the next couple of days I struggled in the tension of opposing choices. Every time I favored a mastectomy, uncertainty nagged me to hang in there and honor my doubts until the deadline for deciding arrived.

In the midst of my perplexity, my trusted friend Belleruth called. I told her which way I was leaning. In return, she asked me what it might feel like to *sacrifice* a part of my body when I didn't have to.

Sacrifice—what a powerful word. Sitting at my computer, I began a conversation with my breast to see what she thought about a mastectomy. I typed in a question and then waited. "I would miss you," she had me type in reply. "I would also feel that you're punishing me—that you believe I intentionally grew this tumor. Caren, I'm shocked to find it here, too." She also assured me that overall I was in excellent health and that we had many more years of life together. When she finished, I thanked her. Then, standing before a full-length mirror, I stripped off my clothes and surveyed my body—front and back. As I went to put my tee shirt back on, I again looked at my breasts and knew without a doubt that I would have a lumpectomy.

■

AFFIRMATION

For the sake of my health, I will retain the courage
of my doubts as well as my convictions.

■

Great doubts deep wisdom. Small doubts little wisdom.
CHINESE PROVERB

O thou of little faith, wherefore didst thou doubt?
MATTHEW 14:31

DREAMS

a visionary creation of the imagination

■

Hold fast to dreams, for if dreams die,
life is a broken-winged bird that cannot fly.
LANGSTON HUGHES

The future belongs to those who believe
in the beauty of their dreams.
ELEANOR ROOSEVELT

Dreams are . . . illustrations from the book
your soul is writing about you.
MARSHA NORMAN

A FEW MONTHS AGO, if you asked Grace M. whether or not she'd ever had a dream come true, she might have said she'd just about given up on dreams. After all, once she dreamed of sharing her sunset years with her husband. But Paul died in his early sixties. She also dreamed that both her children would finish college and marry. They did, but Grace's son-in-law contracted HIV/AIDS. Before he died, he infected his wife. Then, two years ago, Grace learned she had an aggressive form of lung cancer. The news vanquished some of her other dreams.

Determined to survive to make her dream of seeing her three-year-old granddaughter grow up come true, Grace underwent radiation and debilitating chemotherapy treatments. As the treatments, one after the other, weakened her, she found it difficult to breathe without supplemental oxygen. Plastic tubes running from her nose to a metal tank became her steady companions.

Months later, when Grace regained some strength, her friend Helen asked whether she wanted to go to Italy. Without pausing, Grace said, "Yes!" Once abroad, Grace, with the oxygen trailing her, visited a Catholic monastery where a deceased Capuchin monk named Padre Pio once lived. She had met him during a childhood trip to the same town. Now, forty-seven years later, he was a candidate for sainthood.

That night, after leaving the monastery, Grace dreamed that she climbed a very steep flight of stairs and could breathe without using oxygen. Upon reaching the top, she turned and saw Padre Pio standing there. "Is this how you're going to cure me?" she asked. He did not answer. At that point the dream ended. The next morning, after showering, Grace began to straighten up the hotel room.

"What's happened?" Helen asked.

"What do you mean?" Grace answered.

"You're not using oxygen," Helen replied.

On occasion, Grace still uses oxygen—but, she quickly adds, "not like before." Her chest X rays show the cancer is not spreading. "I've never asked for anything," she reflects. "Just that God's will be done. I believe my dream was a sign of what God's will is for me at this time."

■

AFFIRMATION

My dreams can open hidden doors leading to healing and wholeness.

■

Dreams are sent by Zeus.
HOMER

All men of action are dreamers.
PROVERB

EXERCISE

*activity that requires physical or
mental exertion, especially when performed
to develop or maintain fitness*

■

Those who think they have not time for bodily exercise
will sooner or later have to find time for illness.
EDWARD STANLEY

Give your healing system a morning walk and a good night's rest, and it
will be ready for whatever challenges may arise.
ANDREW WEIL

Walking is an excellent exercise. At sixty-five my grandmother began
walking five miles a day. She's now a hundred
and we have no idea where she is.
ELLEN DEGENERES

PREEMINENT AMERICAN HISTORIAN Max Lerner overcame two types
of cancer and then a heart attack before dying in his ninetieth year. In
his last book, *Wrestling with the Angel*, Lerner describes how the walking reg-
imen that he began two years after his heart attack helped to change his negative mood and heal his body.

On his daily walks, Lerner says, he digested the day's ideas and writing
and planned out his work for the morrow. "I carried my current workbook
with me, and I would plot out (in the Yeats phrase) 'what was past and passing and to come' in my workbook and my universe." After awhile, he felt a
"growing serenity within" and found it natural to begin working out in a
gym. To his delight, he discovered that the gym, with "its assemblage of
ingenious contrivances for reinvigorating every muscle and tendon," was

becoming a kind of "machine for living." Gradually, he stepped up the weights for chest, legs, and back and added workouts with a stationary bicycle and punching bag. No matter what else filled his busy days, Lerner always made time for his workout—early morning, late afternoon, sometimes late evening. Over time, exercise became a ritual from which he reaped many unexpected benefits. At age eighty-six, Lerner recorded this journal entry:

My (bone) scan shows some remarkable skeletal improvement, a new "vibrant equilibrium." If he (Dr. Stanley Goldsmith) were studying it without knowing me he would call it the skeleton of a forty-year-old. He says, "we don't understand why this happens, but there it is." I honor his professional humility. But my own guess is that it's the months of workouts with my machines of healing. I am tempted to indite a Hymn to the Gymn.

■

AFFIRMATION

Whenever I take time to exercise, I perform a healing ritual.

■

Exercise expels the superfluities in the body.
MAIMONIDES

It is remarkable how one's wits are sharpened by physical exercise.
PLINY THE YOUNGER

FAITH

*belief that does not rest on logical proof
or material evidence*

■

Faith is the strength by which a shattered world
shall emerge into the light.
HELEN KELLER

Faith is not patience which passively suffers until the storm is passed. It
is rather a spirit which bears things—with resignation, yes, but above all
with blazing, serene hope.
CORAZON AQUINO

Faith is a path of heart that enables us to perceive the mysterious
meaning of life, to confront and overcome obstacles, live with doubt
and paradox, and to be at home in a world where the
Ground of Being is always present.
FREDERIC AND MARY ANN BRUSSAT

I'VE READ A lot of instruction manuals that tell me what other people
have said about losing and finding their faith. However, I'm not so sure
that it's ever really lost. Instead, I've come to believe that faith just gets mis-
placed. Then, when something critical happens that makes us want to hold
onto or keep our faith, we look around saying, "Oy! When did I last have it?"
and begin frantically searching for it like a bunch of missing keys.

For some, the search may lead to a church, synagogue, or some other
spiritual home. For others, searching may mean praying harder and harder,
or trying harder and harder, or looking harder and harder as though those
actions could somehow make the desired outcome manifest. However, if we
think about all the keys that seem to get lost right under our noses, we also

know that it's only when we give up the search that they seem to magically appear.

Breast cancer taught me a lot about faith. First, that I must be willing to let go of outcomes, yet remain hopeful that at the end of my darkness there will be a dawn. Next, I must live in the tension of what I can physically, emotionally, and/or mentally make happen and that which I must be willing to just let happen. For me, that tension meant faithfully taking responsibility for what I could do to help self-heal myself on one hand, while simultaneously placing faith in the love, support, skill, and beneficence of my relatives, friends, doctors, and God on the other.

The word *amen*, which means "It is so," or, "So be it," is found in more than 1,000 languages. Some consider this affirmation of a benediction, prayer, or good wishes to be the most widely used word in human speech. From the time I found a suspicious lump in my breast until I was given a clean bill of health I discovered a missing key to my faith was three simple words patiently waiting to be found in my heart and on the tip of my tongue—*So be it*.

■

AFFIRMATION

So be it.

■

**Faith is confirmed by the heart, confessed by the tongue,
and acted upon by the body.**
SUFI PROVERB

The strength of the heart comes from the soundness of the faith.
ARABIAN PROVERB

FEELINGS

an affective state of consciousness, such as that resulting from emotions, sentiments, or desires

■

Feelings are everywhere—be gentle.
J. MASAI

Never apologize for showing feeling. Remember that when you do so you apologize for truth.
BENJAMIN DISRAELI

He who feels it, knows it more.
BOB MARLEY

BECAUSE I GREW up in a family that discounted feelings, I didn't know I had any until I was an adult. When I hurt, my father would shout, "Stop crying." When I laughed too loud or long, he would ridicule me in a demeaning way. If I expressed anger, I was punished, and if I was "caught" doing a child's random act of kindness, my father usually sneered that I was wasting my time. "Don't bother," he would say. "No one cares."

With so many feelings dulled by my demigod's disapproval of them, I never learned when or where it was appropriate to express them. For example, throughout my childhood, I got lots of cavities. When it came time for my dentist to fill them, I always refused novocaine. Instead, I'd just get a death grip on his chair and signal him to drill away. Once, he pulled one of my teeth without numbing the nerve first. My father was so proud of me for bearing all that pain that he bragged about it. Not until years later did I understand how strange his badge of courage was.

When we push our feelings deep inside, they harden us, instead of helping to heal us. But intuitively, we know they're there, and through unconscious attempts to make the invisible visible, we may turn to self-destructive behaviors. For years, I wouldn't just bite my nails, I would also peel away the layers of thick skin around them and study my raw wounds as if they were maps of my inner world. When I touched them, they'd bleed, sting, and, like my dentist's drill, remind me I was alive. Despite the fact that I knew my hands always looked as if they had gone through a meat grinder, I couldn't stop that self-destructive cycle.

Not until I began peeling back the hardened layers of my psyche and soul instead of the callused skin on my hands was I able to begin to access my repressed feelings. In the process, I rediscovered joy, wonder, happiness, ecstasy, and self-love and found appropriate ways to display anger, grief, sorrow, disappointment, and fear. Most importantly, I also learned what forgiveness felt like. And not long afterwards, a day came when that new feeling stirred me to forgive my father. And when I did, I felt my heart expand and my hands began to heal.

■

AFFIRMATION

My feelings help me to discover my truth and heal my wounds.

■

If you wish me to weep, you must first feel grief.
HORACE

Seeing is believing, but feeling is naked truth.
PROVERB

FLOW

to move or run smoothly with unbroken continuity, as in the manner characteristic of a fluid

■

There's no other flight out tonight—so what?
I'll be an hour late for my meeting if I take a morning flight—so what? I
may blow the deal—so what?
ROBERT RINGER

She had believed the land was her enemy, and she struggled against it,
but you could not make war against a land any more than you could
against the sea. One had to learn to live with it, to belong to it, to fit
into its seasons and its ways.
LOUIS L'AMOUR

Ride the horse in the direction that it's going.
WERNER ERHARD

I N 1974, RENOWNED neurologist and author Oliver Sacks, M.D., had an unfortunate encounter with a bull on a mountain in Norway and severely injured his leg. In *A Leg to Stand On*, Sacks describes the medical journey he took, not as a physician, but as a patient traveling a healing path.

After surgeons repaired his leg, Sacks became terrified by the thought of learning to walk again. On his first day of physical therapy, he had no idea where his left leg was and compared the lifeless limb to a "lump of jelly."

Despite his physiotherapists' efforts to help him take just one step, Sacks's fears immobilized him. When, at last, he clumsily succeeded, he called his robotic motion "unanimal," "unhuman." "Will I never get back the *feel* of true walking . . . which is natural, spontaneous, and free?" he wondered.

His answer came in a moment of grace. In his mind, Sacks heard a beloved Mendelssohnian melody playing and he began walking, easily, joyfully, *with* the music. "In the very moment that my 'motor' music, my kinetic melody, my walking, came back—in this self-same moment *the leg came back.* Suddenly, with no warning, no transition whatever, the leg felt alive, and real, and mine, its moment of actualization precisely consonant with the spontaneous quickening, walking and music."

Describing the exhilaration he felt when he just let go and fell into the rhythm, tempo, pulsation, and feel of walking instead of calculating and mechanically trying to perform each step, Sacks recalled other, less spectacular, times he knew that feeling. "The experience was so common I had hardly given it a thought, but now, I suddenly realized, the experience was fundamental. . . . Everything was transformed, absolutely, in that moment, in that leap from a cold fluttering and flashing to the warm stream of music, the stream of action, the stream of life."

You are the music
While the music lasts
T.S. ELIOT

AFFIRMATION

Going with the flow places me in the stream of life.

Follow the river and you'll get to the sea.
FRENCH PROVERB

Life is a series of natural and spontaneous changes.
Don't resist them . . . .
Let things flow naturally forward in whatever way they like.
LAO-TZU

FORGIVENESS

the act of forgiving; pardon

∎

To forgive is to transform what we would otherwise reject.
MARION WOODMAN

Forgiveness is the answer to the child's dream of a miracle
by which what is broken is made whole again,
what is soiled is again made clean.
DAG HAMMARSKJÖLD

Forgiveness is not to do away with the problem of evil
but to admit its existence and by including it to have
an opportunity of transforming it.
ELIZABETH BOYDEN HOWES

WE ALL KNOW that forgiving oneself and others for mistakes, hurts, and other painful transgressions can have a positive impact on the way old wounds heal. But have you ever considered the role of *unforgiveness*—the opposite of forgiveness—in the healing process?

Psychologist Everett Worthington, a leading voice in the field of forgiveness, says *unforgiveness* refers to a jumble of negative emotions that people feel when someone has hurt them. He knows these emotions well. Shortly after publishing a book on forgiveness, his mother was brutally murdered. "I had to decide whether what I had written was for other people or if I could use it too," he admitted.

The negative emotions associated with unforgiveness can include bitterness, resentment, hostility, anger, hatred, and fear. "Most people," he explains, "think that forgiveness is that thing you do to get rid of unforgiveness, but it turns out there are probably twenty-five things you can do to get rid of unforgiveness without forgiving."

To truly forgive, one must replace the inner negative emotions of unforgiveness with positive, other-oriented emotions. These include love, compassion, and empathy. "Forgiveness is something I grant, so it's an emotional process within me," he says. Furthermore, forgiveness does not occur until we experience a transformation from the negative to the positive. For example, until love or compassion replace anger, there is no forgiveness.

When we forgive another, our entire emotional orientation toward the person who hurt us changes. "That change will filter into your behavior and brain biochemistry, your facial expressions, body posture, and daily life, any time you think about or have to deal with that person," says Worthington, who uses an acronym to REACH forgiveness.

R—Recall the hurt and acknowledge that a wrong was done to you. Set your sights on repair of the wrong.

E—Empathize with the person who hurt you by trying to understand his or her motivations.

A—Altruism: give the gift of forgiveness.

C—Commit to forgiveness.

H—Hold on to forgiveness.

■

AFFIRMATION

I feel kind and generous when I forgive myself and others
for past mistakes and disappointments.

■

To forgive is beautiful.
GREEK PROVERB

To understand is to forgive.
FRENCH PROVERB

FUTURE

the indefinite time yet to come;
something that will happen in times to come

■

Every thought we think is creating our future.
LOUISE HAY

The future influences the present just as much as the past.
FRIEDRICH NIETZSCHE

And I have promises to keep
And miles to go before I sleep.
ROBERT FROST

IN TED'S WORK it's not unusual for him to be called to visit a dying person only to find that his parishioner has rallied—determined to stay alive for a future event. Upcoming birthdays, holidays, graduations, births, marriages, anniversaries, trips, and visits by loved ones are all occasions that have seemingly held an impending death at bay. Similarly, we've all read newspaper accounts of elderly couples who have died on the same day. She passes away because of an accident or illness. Then he dies unexpectedly, because, friends and relatives report, "he had nothing left to live for."

In the spring of 1999, when my seventy-nine-year-old father-in-law learned that a progressive and rare congestive heart condition would claim his life in two to three months, his first words to his wife were, "If I can't go to England, I might as well die right now." For more than two decades, Ed and Millie would travel to the British Isles every fall. There they would spend a month taking workshops to advance their careers as professional artists and enjoy leisurely visits with beloved friends. Now, with Ed barely able to walk ten steps without stopping to rest, making the long journey abroad seemed impossible.

Upon overhearing Ed's comment, his specialist mentioned that he might be a candidate for a clinical trial. "Unfortunately, this drug won't extend your life. However, it has improved the quality of the lives of five patients already taking it." The news made Ed and Millie feel as if they had just snagged the brass ring on a merry-go-round, and even before the drug could actually kick in, his condition began improving. To Ed's delight, by September he felt well enough to travel from North Carolina to Yorkshire and paint at the seashore.

They returned home with lots of stories, sketches, and watercolors. However, within days, Ed's condition began deteriorating. Three weeks later, lying in a coma, he died—not early in the day when the doctors expected him to pass away, but in the late hour when all of his children finally arrived at the hospital to gather at his bedside and lovingly say "Goodbye."

AFFIRMATION

I have promises to myself to keep—now and in the future.

He who foretells the future lies, even if he tells the truth.
ARAB PROVERB

When men speak of the future, the Gods laugh.
CHINESE PROVERB

GIFTS

something given to show friendship,
affection, support, etc.

■

Giving presents is a talent, to know what a person wants, to know when
and how to get it, to give it lovingly and well.
PAMELA GLENCONNER

The only gift is a portion of thyself.
RALPH WALDO EMERSON

I look upon life as a gift from God. I did nothing to earn it.
Now that the time is coming to give it back, I have no right to complain.
JOYCE CARY

WHAT MAKES A gift a gift? I've often wondered. Is it when someone
presents a present to another? Does it have to be intentionally given,
or can it be unconsciously imparted? Is a gift a gift when something given
changes hands? Or is it when the recipient feels gratitude in her heart, not
just her mind, for something that's come her way with no strings attached?
Does our acceptance of a gift return another to the giver? What does a gift
obligate me to—especially this mysterious gift from the Divine called Life?

The first time Ted and I met my surgeon, Ed Staren, M.D., Ph.D., head of
the Cancer Institute at Medical College of Ohio, his broad smile, affable
nature, excellent reputation, and encyclopedic knowledge of his field
bestowed the gift of confidence in him upon us. At that point, we didn't know
whether or not the lump in my breast was malignant. Later, the manner in
which he gave us the bad news reaffirmed the fact that I was not only in good
hands, but in those of a gifted healer.

Before my surgery, Ted and I visited Ed to discuss my options and postoperative treatment. For the first hour, his chief resident, a nurse, and two medical students stood silently as he listened and responded to each of my questions. He then dismissed his entourage and proceeded to spend another hour and a half answering more questions. At the end of each explanation, he would pause to see if either of us wanted more information or if less was enough. He never ended the session. I finally did. And before we left, this man several years my junior gave me a parental hug.

That day, as I received Ed's gifts of wisdom, patience, compassion, and understanding, I reached a new level of self-acceptance and garnered the courage I needed to set foot on the healing path we both designed. Days later, his gifted hands cut into me. Both before and after that moment, Ed's gift of helping me to begin healing changed my life forever.

■

AFFIRMATION

I am grateful for the gifts of healing others may give me
without even knowing it.

■

A gift consists not in what is done or given,
but in the intention of the giver or doer.
SENECA

This also—that I live, I consider a gift of God.
OVID

GRACE

a disposition to be generous or helpful;
mercy; clemency

■

Grace is unity, oneness within ourself, oneness with God.
THOMAS MERTON

Amazing grace!
How sweet the sound,
That saved a wretch like me!
I once was lost, but now I'm found;
Was blind, but now I see.
JOHN NEWTON

In the contemporary idiom, grace is a happening rather than an
achievement, a gift rather than a reward.
SAM KEEN

SOMETHING ABOUT OPERA singer Jessye Norman's rendition of
"Amazing Grace" really gets to me. Whenever I listen to it, I feel compelled
to turn the volume up as loud as I can as, though doing so turns me into a
sponge that can absorb every note, nuance, and word.

Echoing the theme of that wonderful hymn are these words by theologian Paul Tillich:

Grace strikes us when we are in great pain and restlessness. It strikes us when
we walk through the dark valley of a meaningless and empty life. It strikes us
when our disgust for our own being, our indifference, our weakness, our hostility, and our lack of direction and composure have become intolerable to us.
It strikes us when, year after year, the longed-for perfection of life does not
appear, when the old compulsions reign within us as they have for decades,

when despair destroys all joy and courage. Sometimes at that moment a wave of light breaks into our darkness, and it is as though a voice were saying: "You are accepted."

In four short verses, "Amazing Grace" expands my understanding of Tillich's words. Listening to the story the words tell about the captain of a slave ship who suddenly understands that his cargo is not a commodity but a sea of humanity reconnects me with those remarkable times when a wave of healing light has broken my darkness. One such moment occurred when, shortly before my father's death, this abusive, raging man asked for my forgiveness while tearfully telling me about the abuses he, himself, had suffered as a child.

Another was when I looked through a sheer curtain veiling a window and saw my mother sitting peacefully on the swing on my front porch. For most of my life, her addictions had cloaked our relationship. Now, in her twilight years, she was alcohol and drug free and full of laughter and love. As I stood staring at this gossamer blonde angel, I suddenly saw beyond all my mother had never been to me and could at last accept and feel love for who she had become.

Amazing grace! In a flash grace can open our eyes and help heal our blindness to others and ourselves.

■

AFFIRMATION

I am thankful for moments of grace that help heal my wounded and broken relationships.

■

God does not refuse grace to those who do what they can.
LATIN PROVERB

The ideal man bears the accidents of life with dignity and grace, making the best of circumstances.
ARISTOTLE

GRATITUDE

the state of being grateful; thankfulness

◼

Gratitude births only positive feelings—love, compassion, joy, and
hope. As we focus on what we are thankful for, fear, anger, and bitterness simply melt away, seemingly without effort.
M.J. RYAN

Gratitude unlocks the fullness of life. It turns what we have into
enough, and more. It turns denial into acceptance, chaos to order, confusion to clarity. Gratitude makes sense of our past, brings peace for
today, and creates a vision for tomorrow.
MELODY BEATTIE

To speak gratitude is courteous and pleasant, to enact gratitude is generous and noble, to live gratitude is to touch heaven.
JOAHANNES A. GAERTNER

ACCORDING TO AN old *Saturday Evening Post* story, the Pilgrims had a cus-
tom of putting five grains of corn on each empty plate before a dinner
of "thanksgiving" was served. Then those gathered around the table would
each take turns picking up their grains and telling their family and friends
about something for which they were thankful. "The practice reminded
them of how the first Pilgrims were in such straits that their allowance was
only five grains of corn per person each day," the article said. "The Pilgrims
had little, but they did possess gratitude."

I find it interesting that ultimately the English word for "thanks" arose out
of Indo-European words for "think" and "thoughtfulness." Although I know
there are times when I thoughtlessly say "Thank you" in response to another's words or deeds, my sincerest expressions of gratitude are more thought
filled. For example, over the years, I've made it a practice occasionally to

stop and think of people in my past who unselfishly bestowed healing gifts of time, energy, presence, trust, confidence, truth, and love upon me. I then try to express my gratitude through letters, cards, phone calls, visits, deeds, or donations in their honor. Recipients of these tokens have been relatives, mentors, friends, and even strangers.

Several years ago, the phrase "random acts of kindness" became popular. Many of these acts were very small, simple ones that made a difference in the recipient's life. Professor Rudolph Arnheim tells this story about his lasting gratitude for one such kindness: "At a faculty reception, a British lady taught me how to tie my shoes with a double knot so that they keep tied more securely and still come apart in a jiffy," he said. "Kneeling on the floor in the midst of the chattering sherry-sippers, she tied my shoes. I remember her twice a day ever since."

AFFIRMATION

When I express gratitude to others, I transform my thoughts into deeds.

Praise the bridge that carried you over.
ENGLISH PROVERB

If something that was going to chop off our head only knocked off our cap, we should be grateful.
YORUBA PROVERB

GRIEF

to experience or express grief

■

Grief is itself a med'cine.
WILLIAM COWPER

She was no longer wrestling with the grief, but could sit down with it as
a lasting companion and make it a sharer in her thoughts.
GEORGE ELIOT

No one ever told me that grief felt so like fear.
C.S. LEWIS

THE TWO TIMES when words really fail to describe what we feel are when
we fall in love and when we suffer grief. Recently, a friend whose husband died unexpectedly told me that it took her a long time to acknowledge
her grief. "I kept going through motions instead of *emotions*," she said. A
well-known Buddhist story called "The Mustard Seed" talks about our need
to pay attention to our grief and the healing we experience by giving it
voice.

At the opening of the story, Kisa Gotami, a poor and frail Indian woman,
has finally received some respect after marrying and giving birth to a son.
One day, a swift and fatal illness overcame the child, whom Kisa loved more
than anything else. Crazed with grief over his death, she took her precious
child in her arms and ran from door to door hoping to find someone who
had medicine that could restore his life. But no one could, and many
mocked her for thinking it was possible.

As she stood on the street sobbing, along came a man who took her to see
the Buddha. While looking at the lifeless child's face, the Buddha reassured
Kisa that she was wise to come for medicine. However, before he would give

it to her, the Buddha told her, she must first go throughout the city, find a mustard seed from a family in which no one had died, and bring it back to him.

So the next morning, Kisa again knocked on one door, then another. Each time, she heard the same story. In every household, someone's son, daughter, parent, spouse, aunt, or uncle had died, and the pain and grief the surviving members suffered was beyond words. By twilight, Kisa knew she was not alone.

The next day, Kisa tearfully buried her only child. After the funeral, she returned to the Buddha to tell him she had not found the mustard seed but had learned that no one is free from the certainty of death. She then said, "We must help each other, as you have helped me." And so she did.

> This is the Hour of Lead—
> Remembered, if outlived,
> As Freezing persons, recollect the Snow—
> First—Chill—then Stupor—then the letting go—
> EMILY DICKINSON

■

AFFIRMATION

When I allow myself to feel grief, it expresses what words cannot.

■

Suppressed grief suffocates.
LATIN PROVERB

There is no grief which time does not lessen.
LATIN PROVERB

GROWTH

to allow (something) to develop or
increase by a natural process

■

The art of living lies less in eliminating our troubles
than in growing with them.
BERNARD M. BARUCH

Life is growth. If we stop growing, technically and spiritually,
we are as good as dead.
MORIHEI UESHIBA

Growth begins when we start to accept our weaknesses.
JEAN VANIER

WE NAMED OUR West Virginia home "Berkana," which is an ancient symbol for "growth." In some ways our choice is ironic, since almost all our attempts to plant anything there have been foiled by the deer.

Berkana sits in the midst of a wildlife preserve where hunting or harming animals is forbidden. Therefore, deer ranging in size from tiny Bambis to ten-point bucks roam everywhere and eat almost everything that grows as they cut a swath through vegetation in their path and make liars out of nurserymen who hawk "deerproof" plants. In a deer's wake, daisy stems stand daisyless. Saplings become leafless, barkless twigs, and ground cover disappears like a balding man's hair. Not surprisingly, after years of coexistence, herds of hoofed ruminants have taught us a lot about what it takes to grow in the midst of adversity.

To grow, you must first commit to preparing the ground so it can support the process for a long time. In the beginning, it's necessary to set boundaries, because without them predators, like deer, weeds, and viruses, will go everywhere. To keep intruders at bay, use something that protects, but doesn't smother, whatever is trying to grow. Doing that gives it room to remain grounded and self-heal its wounds even under difficult and life-threatening circumstances. It is also important to realize that not everything that grows and grows well grows up.

Once whatever is growing matures enough to survive alone, it's time to give it responsibility for itself. If you've fostered inner strength and good health, storms and tidal waves may cause it to falter, but those natural events won't be fatal. Additionally, you must become reconciled *to*, not *with*, whatever adversely affects growth. At Berkana, we're never going to be reconciled *with* the deer. They just don't care. However, we can be reconciled *to* their abiding presence. And, finally, turn to other teachers. Take the trees and ground cover, for instance. They've taught us that to mature, be healthy, and heal our wounds, we must grow at our own pace and be willing to move in lots of directions. Occasionally, we must also turn to outside support, not allow open wounds or hidden hurts to fester, be flexible, and respond appropriately to all the seasons of our lives.

■

AFFIRMATION

I am grateful for the resources and people who support my growth.

■

Without bending, there is no growth.
JAPANESE PROVERB

One cannot grow higher than oneself.
RUSSIAN PROVERB

HEAL

to restore to health or soundness;
to become whole and sound

■

Thank God for what doesn't need healing.
JOAN BORYSENKO

Healing, is the intuitive art of wooing Nature.
W.H. AUDEN

The treatment is really a cooperative effort of a trinity—the patient, the
doctor, and the inner doctor.
RALPH BIRCH

M Y FAVORITE HEALING story tells of a paralytic man whose four friends
carry him on a bed to see Jesus. Upon arriving at Jesus's home, they
discover that to get to him they must lower the bed through the roof. When
they do, the writer tells us, Jesus sees their faith and says, "Your sins are forgiven . . . rise, take up your bed and go home." Immediately, the paralytic
rises and goes out. Amazed, the crowd says, "We have seen strange things
today," and praises God.

Although many interpretations place the healing power in Jesus's hands,
the story does not. Nowhere is it reported that Jesus said, "*I* heal you," or "*I*
forgive your sins." So, I wonder, what is it that this first-century Jew adds to
the paralytic's healing equation? Whose faith did Jesus see and what, in fact,
is that faith?

When this story was written, one way that a Jew's sins were forgiven was
by means of a specific sacrificial process. But instead of telling the paralytic
to go that route, Jesus merely tells him that his sins are forgiven—rise. If
that's so, what sacrifices and atonement might the paralytic have made

earlier in order to be healed? Did he sacrifice his pride? Did it cost him financial or other resources? We can only imagine. And, finally, why might one have to take one's bed with one? Why not just leave it behind?

One reason I enjoy this story so much is that it challenges me to revisit my own healing journeys. Who, in the past, have been my helpers? What about now? What role has faith played in restoring the parts of me that get "paralyzed?" What, if anything, must I sacrifice for the sake of healing? If the word *sin* originally meant "missing the mark," how and when have my words or actions missed the mark and forestalled healing? Must I forgive and be forgiven before I can be healed? Is healing something I do for and by myself, or is an outside catalyst always needed? Where and when does healing begin? Does the process ever end?

Novelist Tim O'Brien once said, "Just because it didn't happen doesn't mean it isn't true." I love this story, because even if it didn't happen, my own healing journey tells me that it is definitely true.

■

AFFIRMATION

Today I am grateful for people past and present
who have played a role in my healing journey.

■

The wish for healing has ever been the half of health.
SENECA

Every invalid is a physician.
IRISH PROVERB

HEALTH

a condition of optimal well-being

■

Our health is a voyage and every illness is an adventure story.
MARGIAD EVANS

You already have the precious mixture that will
make you well. Use it.
JALAL-UDDIN RUMI

The healthy individual is the one who asks for help when he needs it.
Whether he has an abscess on his knee or in his soul.
RONA BARRETT

THE HEBREW EXPRESSION *l'chayim* (which, according to Leo Rosten, rhymes with "to fry 'em" and the *ch* sounds as if you're clearing your throat) means "to life." Worldwide, it's used as a toast meaning "To your health." Contained in the word *l'chayim* is another—*chai*—which means "hope for life."

To think about health—be it another's or our own—without thinking about life is virtually impossible. Therefore, I like the idea that most of our thoughts about health contain an unspoken prayer that expresses our "hope for life."

According to the World Health Organization constitution, "Health is a state of complete physical, mental and social well-being, and not merely the absence of disease or infirmity." Anyone who has ever lived with or cared for someone with a chronic or life-threatening illness knows the deepest truths contained in WHO's definition. Whether we're healthy or not, our condition adds up to more than the sum of our parts, because it affects others in our lives as well.

Not too long ago, we got a cross-country call from one of our closest friends. She wanted to tell us that she had "bottomed out"—that she was a drug addict. She realized, she said, that if she didn't enter a three-month residential rehabilitation program, she stood to lose everything—not just her physical health, but her husband and young child, her financial resources, her family's support, her friends, and, perhaps, her life. Although her husband knew that her growing dependency on cocaine threatened the health of their marriage, he lived in denial until the impact of the addiction affecting one of them began to consume both.

Upon hearing her sad news, we offered our love and support and said, "*L'chayim.*" *L'chayim*—a toast to your health, dear friend, because we know that without good health, the world you've helped brighten is clouded in darkness that feels lifeless. *L'chayim*—our hope for your new life, because whenever serious illness or a natural disaster compromises our health, we cannot return to life as we once knew it. *L'chayim*—our prayer that the responsibility that you've chosen to take for your health assures you a healthy, prosperous, and long life. And *l'chayim*—the blessing we offer to you and those who care for and love you as you begin your healing journey.

■

AFFIRMATION

L'chayim!

■

A wise man ought to realize that health
is his most valuable possession.
HIPPOCRATES

Having good health is very different from only being not sick.
SENECA

HEART

*the chambered, muscular organ that maintains
the flow of blood through the entire
circulatory system; the vital center and source of
one's being, emotions, and sensibilities*

■

Though pain may crack the heart open—leaving us raw—rather than taking
something away from us, it offers us a chance to be present to our own life
process, to feel the heart stirrings—even though the pain is there.

HELEN HUNT

A slimy, throbbing mass of muscle entwined in its own veins and arter-
ies, a tender, fearsome instrument of love and power—the heart!

GEORGE LEONARD

There are pains that cannot be contained in the mind—only in the heart.

STEPHEN LEVINE

ONCE UPON A time, Claire Sylvia's view of the heart was similar to that
held by Western medicine. For her, the organ that ancient peoples considered to be the seat of love, courage, the intellect, and the soul was merely a mechanism that carried no wisdom, no knowledge, and no memories.
However, today, Sylvia, who underwent a heart-lung transplant in 1988,
knows otherwise.

Almost immediately after the lifesaving operation that removed her
damaged organs and replaced them with those of an eighteen-year-old man
who had died just hours earlier in a motorcycle accident, Sylvia began to
experience unusual thoughts, cravings, and emotions. In the months that
followed, many of her habits and tastes changed, and she began to intuit that
her new heart had something to do with it. Five months later, Sylvia had a

remarkable dream about a young man named Tim. Upon awakening, she knew that it was his heart that beat in her chest, and she became determined to find his family. After lots of sleuthing, Sylvia finally learned that the anonymous donor was, indeed, named Tim. Moreover, when she met his family, she also discovered that her new and radically different behaviors, thoughts, and emotional responses echoed his.

Reflecting in her memoir, *A Change of Heart*, Sylvia now believes that qualities commonly attributed to the heart are more than metaphorical. "Even today, in our enlightened, scientific era, we still refer to the heart when we discuss our feelings and our values," she says. "When love dies, or death strikes, we speak of being brokenhearted. We take heart and lose heart all the time. When we want to be demonstrative, we wear our heart on our sleeve; when a person is insensitive, we say he is heartless. Pure heart, aching heart, soft heart, valiant heart, noble heart, tender heart, understanding heart—the list goes on." Might there possibly be some literal truth to these expressions, she wonders.

"Although Tim's life was cut short, his spirit, along with his organs, were evidently meant to continue living," says Sylvia. "I believe that he led me to find his family, to be in touch with them again, and perhaps to resolve or complete that which was unresolved while he lived. I feel this strongly in my heart. . . . I feel privileged to be alive."

■

AFFIRMATION

More and more I know that matters of my heart matter.

■

When the heart is at ease, the body is healthy.
CHINESE PROVERB

It's a poor heart that never rejoices.
ENGLISH PROVERB

HOPE

*to look forward to with confidence or expecta-
tion; a wish or desire accompanied by confident
expectation of its fulfillment*

■

In the depth of winter I finally learned
that there was in me an invincible summer.
ALBERT CAMUS

Hope is not the conviction that something will turn out well but the
certainty that something makes sense, regardless of how it turns out.
VÁCLAV HAVEL

There is no medicine like hope, no incentive so great, and no tonic so
powerful as expectation of something tomorrow.
ORISON SWETT MARDEN

HOW MANY TIMES have the words "I hope everything will be okay" tumbled out of your mouth in response to unsettling news? Just yesterday,
they circled in my mind as I learned that the Rev. Bill Dols, one of my dearest friends and mentors, had cancer.

As former breast cancer patients, both Bill's wife, Shirley, and I agreed
we knew what he might have felt upon hearing that dreaded C word.
Confusion, fear, anger, guilt, sorrow, apprehension, anxiety, and emptiness
were all possibilities. But, I knew from experience, hopeful was, too.

Hope, my encounter with cancer taught me, is an attitude that's seated
in our hearts to help us live in the tension between our wishes and desires
on one hand and our disappointments, failures, tragedies, and despair on the
other. Hope, says Benedictine Brother David Steindl-Rast, is openness for

surprise as we stand poised between the already and the not-yet. It is the pilgrim's passion for the possible that "holds the present open for an ever fresh future."

Whenever we pilgrims on the way trip over sickness, loss, and other stumbling blocks, it is hope that bolsters our resolve to search for a healing path. Hope for wellness, vitality, and a better life urges us to move forward into an unknown future with treatments, protocols, requests for help, and other practical responses. Hope sets our hearts and our sights on our goals and sustains our desire to attain them. Hope does not require us to be optimists *instead* of pessimists. It just asks that even in our most cynical moments we do not shut the door to a "fresh future."

While waiting for Bill to tell me what his doctors had told him about his cancer, I hoped his healing path would be gentle. "They got everything and I won't need radiation or chemo," he told me later. "However, I have to go back in four months. They want to see if it returns. . . ."

We must accept finite disappointment, but we must never lose infinite hope.
REV. MARTIN LUTHER KING, JR.

■

AFFIRMATION

My hope sets my heart and my sights on goals that help heal me.

■

Hope is the last thing ever lost.
ITALIAN PROVERB

Hope holds up the head.
SCOTTISH PROVERB

HUMOR

the ability to perceive, enjoy, or express what is
amusing, comical, incongruous, or absurd

■

Humor is emotional chaos remembered in tranquility.
JAMES THURBER

You can turn painful situations around through laughter. If you can find
humor in anything—even poverty—you can survive it.
BILL COSBY

Cancer is probably the most unfunny thing in the world,
but I'm a comedienne, and even cancer couldn't stop me from
seeing humor in what I went through.
GILDA RADNER

THE LATE *New York Times* drama critic Brooks Atkinson said that humor is
not merely the telling of funny stories. "It recognizes the vast difference
between life as we imagine it and life as we live it, and between the fanciful
and imposing impressions we have of ourselves and what we actually are."

Illness always forces us to live some aspects of our lives in ways we had
never imagined. Not surprisingly, at those times our only certainty may be
that we feel uncertain about our future. Humorist Steve Bhaerman, who
writes and performs as his alter ego, Swami Beyondananda, believes that
humor helps us develop the flexibility we need to find new ways of seeing
our world and dealing with uncertainty. "A good paradoxical joke can wres-
tle the mind to the ground and allow surrender to a deeper reality."

Whether he's writing or performing, the swami directs most of his
energies toward helping people to learn the Chinese healing practice of Fu
Ling and discover the farce is with them. "Four out of five metaphysicians

recommend levity as the best way to rise above the gravity of whatever is bringing you down." As he sees it, duck soup, a hearty laughingstock anyone can make from his or her own ingredients, is one of the best balms for making people explode with laughter. "Humor helps to heal our minds, bodies, and spirits because it helps us milk the sacred cow and render the bull harmless."

Although the swami never guarantees that we will reach our fool potential, he does believe all of us have the ability to open our clown chakras, activate our farce field, and increase our laugh expectancy. "Life is a joke, but God is laughing with us, not at us," he explains. "In a universe that's a friendly place, we take turns being comedian and straight man so we get the fool spectrum of experience. FUNdamentalists are ardently pro-laugh and pro-choice. If you want to be miserable go right ahead—whatever makes you happy."

AFFIRMATION

Whenever I open my clown chakra and activate my farce field,
I increase my laugh expectancy.

Many a true word is spoken in jest.
ENGLISH PROVERB

A merry heart doeth good like medicine.
PROVERBS

IMAGINATION

the ability to confront and deal with reality by
using the creative power of the mind; resource-
fulness

■

Imagination is the voice of daring. If there is anything Godlike about
God it is that. He dared to imagine everything.
HENRY MILLER

There is neither beginning nor end to the imagination but it delights in
its own seasons reversing the usual order at will.
WILLIAM CARLOS WILLIAMS

Use your imagination not to scare yourself to death
but to inspire yourself to life.
ADELE BROOKMAN

IN HER INSIGHTFUL book *Good Grief: Healing through the Shadow of Loss,*
Deborah Morris Coryell challenges her readers to embrace loss. Coryell,
the cofounder and executive director of the Shiva Foundation, an organization dedicated to offering resources and support to people dealing with loss
and death, knows the subject intimately. In 1981, a tumor on her throat
proved to be metastatic thyroid cancer. As a result, she became fascinated by
what she calls the metaphorical equivalence of disease—the idea that illness
does not arbitrarily come into our lives. Instead, it is a function of how we
care for, think, and feel about ourselves.

Intrigued by a statement by psychologist Carl Jung that healing lives in
the realm of the imaginal, Coryell pondered the role our minds play in the
healing process. "What exactly is 'the realm of the imaginal?' " she asked

herself. Then, answering her own question, Coryell concluded, "The imaginal lives in what we see with our imagination, the vision of the mind's eye. Most of us have grown up in a culture where the imagination has been grossly underrated. If you want to invalidate a friend's feelings you tell them what they are feeling is 'just their imagination,' or respond with, 'it's all in your mind,' to someone's fears. But our minds are all we've got. The imagination lets a blind person see; the imagination is where dreams are born; the imagination is where healing begins."

For Coryell, healing is the act of remembering ourselves back into wholeness after we've been dismembered. It can begin several different ways—as a thought, as an idea, or as a picture in our minds. "Healing in the realm of the imaginal means looking at the images we have in our minds; listening to the thoughts with which we are obsessed; hearing the words that are coming out of our mouths and making a conscious decision to have thoughts and images, and speak words that bring us back into wholeness. . . . Healing lives in the images with which we choose to live."

■

AFFIRMATION

Healing lives in the images with which I choose to live.

■

The eyes are not responsible when the mind does the seeing.
PUBILIUS SYRUS

We are what we think. With our thoughts, we make our world.
THE BUDDHA

IMMORTALITY

the quality or condition of being immortal; end-less life or existence

■

Our Creator would never have made such lovely days and have given
us the deep hearts to enjoy them unless we were meant to be immortal.
NATHANIEL HAWTHORNE

Something began me and it had no beginning: something will end me
and it has no end.
CARL SANDBURG

We feel and know that we are eternal.
BENEDICT SPINOZA

THE NEWS THAT I had cancer caused an abiding fear of dying to kick me
in the gut. It was a painful reminder that, no matter how many times
I've told myself that death would not have dominion over me, my fear of not
dying a good death was quite another issue. Not surprisingly, the fact that I
had a life-threatening illness pushed me to wonder again whether there's life
after death. I have only to look at my seven-year-old granddaughter, Andie,
to find an answer.

Andie looks almost exactly like her mother, Jamie. My daughter, Jamie,
I have always been told, looks "exactly" like me. Though after thirty-one
years I still find it hard to see the resemblance, strangers in supermarket
checkout lines say we're cloned. I admit that sometimes, when I look at
Jamie, I see a mannerism that she could only have gotten from me. Could it
be our walks, our smiles, the tilt of our heads reside in ancient DNA that
has passed from generation to generation? It reminds me of the first time I

looked in the mirror and saw my mother's face staring back or said something to my children and realized it wasn't me speaking, but she.

Now that my mother has died, I've become more aware of what immortality might really mean. When I do something to honor her memory, I keep alive her goodness, compassion, generosity, and juiciness, and possibly her attributes on the other side of that equation, too. When I tell Andie stories about her great nana, she's apt to shed tears of remembrance. When I ask her, "Why so sad?" she tells me that my mother is in her heart and it really hurts because she can only feel her but not see her, too. My heart agrees.

"I want to go on living even after my death," wrote Anne Frank shortly before she perished in the Holocaust. Today, more than fifty years later, we know that every time someone reads Frank's diary, it immortalizes this courageous twelve-year-old in his or her heart. Looking at Andie, I have no doubt that I, too, am immortal.

■

AFFIRMATION

I am grateful for the gift of life—now and forever.

■

These bodies are perishable; but the dwellers in these bodies are eternal, indestructible, and impenetrable.
BHAGAVAD-GITA

He who knows that this body is like froth, and has learnt that it is as unsubstantial as a mirage, will break the flower-pointed arrow of Mara, and never see the king of death.
DHAMMAPADA

INTUITION

*the act or faculty of knowing or sensing
without the use of rational processes;
immediate cognition*

■

It is always with excitement that I wake up in the morning wondering
what my intuition will toss up to me, like gifts from the sea. I work with
it and rely on it. It's my partner.
JONAS SALK

The only real valuable thing is intuition.
ALBERT EINSTEIN

Intuition is no big deal. Everybody has it. The good news, for those who
consider themselves highly intuitive—you're not weird; the bad news:
you're not special either.
BELLERUTH NAPARSTEK

FOUR CENTURIES AGO, Phillipus Aureolus Theophrastus Bombost von Hohenheim (Paracelsus), the great German-Swiss physician, held that intuition was "necessary to understand the patient, his body, his disease." Within a hundred years that qualifying principle disappeared as the practice of medicine became a strict, scientific endeavor. Today, as most physicians continue to ignore the value intuition may have in the healing equation, some, such as Mike Marcotte, an obstetrician specializing in high-risk pregnancies, are choosing to factor it back in.

While most obstetricians deliver good news to expectant parents, that's not the norm for Mike. Often it's his job to be the bearer of bad news, the dasher of dreams. "That's where I've really learned to trust my intuition along with my scientific training," he says. "When a mother learns that something is wrong and that her child may have very serious problems or not be able to sustain life after birth, it is devastating. That's when I listen for a voice inside that can tell me what I need to do to help guide her through a dark time and place."

Although medical school never taught Mike how to use his sixth sense, he believes it's a priceless tool available to all of us.

"I can't explain my experience physiologically, but I know I couldn't practice medicine without it. As physicians we wish to do no harm. But knowing what does harm is not just about following laws, rules and procedures. It's also about matters of the heart and soul and being patient, compassionate, and aware. My goal is to always try to help parents step onto a healing path that can lead them through their disappointment and grief. The only way I can find the thoughts and words to do that is to go deep inside and tap into instincts that know more about those matters than my conscious self does. When I'm willing to trust that process, I always learn something about healing—and myself—that medical school could never teach me."

■

AFFIRMATION

More and more I am learning to listen to and trust
the healing words my intuition offers me.

■

A good artist lets his intuition lead him wherever it wants.
LAO-TZU

Spend time every day listening to what your
muse is trying to tell you.
SAINT BARTHOLOMEW

JOURNALING

the act of recording one's thoughts

■

I want to write, but more than that,
I want to bring out all kinds of things that lie buried in my heart.
ANNE FRANK

To write "my body" plunges me into lived experience, particularity.
I see scars, disfigurements, discolorations, damages, losses,
as well as what pleases me.
ADRIENNE RICH

"Journaling provides an ongoing record of one's
therapeutic progress. Months and years later, your journal
offers documentation and assurance that as time passes,
wounds heal and circumstances change."
KATHLEEN ADAMS

ON CHRISTMAS EVE in 1993 in Toledo, Ohio, Laurie Hoeffel's thirty-four-year-old son Rick lay dying of AIDS. This was hardly a silent night, as the oldest of her eight children labored to breathe, lost control of his bowels, and moaned from his pain. Love and duty intermingled as she nursed him, until finally Rick became comfortable enough to sleep. Sighing from exhaustion and the realization that her husband, other children, and grandchildren were all gathered around their Christmas tree two miles away, Laurie settled into a chair next to her son's bed. She lit a votive candle, then began confessing her innermost thoughts, questions, and feelings to the only companion she trusted completely—her journal.

An hour later, Laurie put down her pen, closed her spiral-bound notebook, and tucked it away for safekeeping. Soon a hospice nurse would relieve her, and she would return home with this record of her journey, brimming with reflections about a period of her life she never could have imagined three years earlier.

"Thank goodness for my journal," Laurie said later. "For twenty years it's been my therapist. It never judges me for my thoughts. Instead it helps me clarify them. My journal is a mirror that honestly reflects everything I think, feel, and experience. At times it knows things about me that I don't even know about myself." In the best-selling book *The Artist's Way*, author Julia Cameron says that when we discipline ourselves to write three strictly stream of consciousness pages every morning, it's analogous to prayer. There's no right or wrong way to do this, she says. But when we do, these pages become a pathway to a strong and clear sense of self that helps us to map our own interior.

Like many people who keep both written and tape-recorded journals, Laurie fills hers with events, ideas, decisions, dreams, observations, and sorrows. Sometimes she paints a thought or a dream; sometimes she pastes in a token or remembrance of a place. When she periodically rereads her journals, Laurie believes that a trustworthy voice bent on helping her to grow emotionally and spiritually is speaking to her. "Journaling," she concludes, "is a healing gift that I give to myself."

■

AFFIRMATION

When I take time to journal, I give voice to my psyche and soul.

■

Write down all these things that have happened to you.
TOBIAS 12:20

This is the dream that you saw. . . . Therefore write all these things that
you have seen in a book, put it in a hidden place.
2 ESDRAS 12:35

JOURNEY

*the act of traveling from one place to another; a
process or course likened to traveling*

■

No traveler e'er reached that blest abode
who found not thorns and briers in his road.
WILLIAM COWPER

If you want to catch beasts you don't see everyday,
You have to go places quite out-of-the-way.
You have to go places no others can get to.
You have to get cold, and you have to get wet, too.
DR. SEUSS

It is good to have an end to journey toward,
but it is the journey that matters in the end.
URSULA K. LEGUIN

"FOLLOW THE YELLOW brick road. Follow the yellow brick road." At the
beginning of Dorothy's journey through the Land of Oz, she believed
that all she had to do to get back home was to follow the yellow brick road
to a wonderful wizard who could magically send her back to Kansas.

As we soon find out, the road Dorothy must travel to get to the wizard
is not smooth. She encounters a lion, flying monkeys, and other scary creatures. Sometimes her helpmates on the way become problematic. Near the
end of her journey, when she needs to be particularly mindful of every
move, Dorothy and her buddies become intoxicated and unconscious in a
poppy field. And finally, after reaching the end of the road, the intrepid and
courageous Dorothy finds that the wizard she pinned her hopes on isn't so
wonderful. He can't do a thing to mend her life. Only she has the power to
do that, says a good witch.

Whenever illness, divorce, death, losing a job, or some other devastating whirlwind lifts us out of our familiar surroundings and hurls us over the rainbow into a foreign land, we resonate with Dorothy's journey. Upon landing, we feel frightened, shaky, disoriented, and unsure about where to turn next. Others—doctors, lawyers, consultants, clergy, friends, and relatives—can offer advice and point us toward a healing path. But no matter what directions or reassurances they give, we're the ones who must summon the courage to take the first step. Because we've no experience travelling this road, we're unaware of stumbling blocks, dead-ends, and all the deep, dark places that we're destined to visit before arriving on the other side. Then, when we finally do get there, we, like Dorothy, may discover that others—even our best wizards—cannot change our lives. The healing changes we courageously sought for our bodies, minds, and spirits must come from within. But now, thanks to our journeys, we do, at last, have the wisdom, strength, determination, perspective, and belief in ourselves to choose to make them happen.

■

AFFIRMATION

My journey to self-healing begins with my courage to take the first step.

■

You can only go halfway into the darkest forest;
then you are coming out the other side.
CHINESE PROVERB

A good traveller has no fixed plans and is not intent upon arriving.
LAO-TZU

JOY

*the intense and especially ecstatic or exultant
happiness; great pleasure; rejoicing*

■

Sometimes your joy is the source of your smile,
but sometimes your smile can be the source of your joy.
THICH NHAT HANH

When you finally allow yourself to trust joy and embrace it,
you will find you dance with everything.
EMMANUEL

Health is not just the absence of a disease. It's an inner joyfulness that
should be ours all the time—a state of positive well-being.
DEEPAK CHOPRA

IN 1984, TWO weeks before her fiftieth birthday and six years after having a mastectomy, Black lesbian feminist, warrior, mother, poet, essayist,
educator, and activist Audre Lorde learned she now had liver cancer. Her
doctors gave her only three to five years to live. Defiantly, Audre died
almost eight years later, on November 17, 1992. Her last book, *A Burst of
Light*, contains an essay by the same name that describes her healing journey. To all those who have ever been told their days are measured, Lorde
offers these wise words about how one can choose to live them joyously.

I believe that one of the ways in which cancer cells insure their own life and
depress the immune system is by creating a physiologically engendered
despair. Learning to fight that despair in its manifestations is not only therapeutic. It is vital. Underlying what is joyful and life-affirming in my living
becomes crucial.

One of the hardest things to accept is learning to live within uncertainty and neither deny it nor hide behind it. Most of all, to listen to the messages of uncertainty without allowing them to immobilize me, nor keep me from the certainties of those truths in which I believe. . . . This is my life. Each hour is a possibility not to be banked. These days are not a preparation for living, some necessary but essentially extraneous divergence from the main course of my living. They are my life.

. . . An open-eyed assessment and appreciation of what I can and do accomplish, using who I am and who I most wish myself to be. To stretch as far as I can go and relish what is satisfying rather than what is sad.

I work, I love, I rest, I see and learn. And I report. These are my givens. Not sureties, but a firm belief that whether or not living them with joy prolongs my life, it certainly enables me to pursue the objectives of that life with a deeper and more effective clarity.

■

AFFIRMATION

When I embrace life I've been given with joy, I affirm all that is life-giving.

■

One joy scatters a hundred griefs.
CHINESE PROVERB

No earthly joy is acquired without tears.
PHILLIPINE PROVERB

LAUGHTER

the act of laughing;
the sound produced by laughing

■

Seven days without laughter makes one weak.
JOEL GOODMAN

I have seen what a laugh can do. It can transform almost
unbearable tears into something bearable, even hopeful.
BOB HOPE

Laughter restores the universe to its original state of indifference and
strangeness: if it has a meaning, it is a divine one,
not a human one.
OCTAVIO PAZ

ALTHOUGH SOCIAL SCIENTISTS have yet to figure out why our Creator graced us with the gift of laughter, who among us could imagine exchanging this precious response to the human condition for something else? Thanks to the late Norman Cousins, whose best-selling book *Anatomy of an Illness* described how a daily dose of laughter helped cure his life-threatening disease, we're now very aware that guffaws, chuckles, cackles, and other expressions of glee positively affect blood pressure, heart rate, and stress. Indeed, recent studies show that ten minutes of hearty ha-ha-ing equates with thirty minutes to an hour of meditation.

Like *Reader's Digest* and the Bible, Cousins called laughter "the best medicine." It's a form of internal jogging that moves our internal organs around, enhances respiration, and ignites great expectations, he said. I have no doubt. I remember that shortly after I learned I had cancer, I began mentally making a list of my favorite stand-up comedians. My doctors said I would need thirty-three radiation treatments, and if that was the case, Jerry

Seinfeld, Bill Cosby, Stephen Wright, Bob Newhart, and others would drive back and forth with me. Daily, each took turns helping me to lighten up, breathe more heartily, and sometimes release hidden tears.

I guess that's really one of the strangest things about laughter—that as it ripples along a continuum of emotions, it can move us to tears. Journalist Linda Ellerbee, who often talks about her breast cancer, believes that laughter may actually be a form of courage. "As humans we sometimes stand tall and look into the sun and laugh, and I think we are never more brave than when we do that."

According to Frederic and Mary Ann Brussat, authors and editors of *Spiritual Literacy*, an Apache myth tells of the Creator giving human beings the ability to talk, to run, and to look. But not until the Creator gave them the ability to laugh could he say, "Now you are fit to live." Mary Pettibone Poole sums up the healing power of laughter this way: "He who laughs, lasts."

■

AFFIRMATION

Each time I go "Ha, ha," my body goes, "Aaaahhhh."

■

**A good laugh and a long sleep
are the best cures in the doctor's book.**
IRISH PROVERB

What soap is to the body, laughter is to the soul.
YIDDISH PROVERB

LIBERATE

to set free, as from oppression, confinement

◼

Your pain is the breaking of the shell that
encloses your understanding.
KAHLIL GIBRAN

To see your drama clearly is to be liberated from it.
KEN KEYES

Begin to free yourself at once by doing all that is possible
with the means you have, and as you proceed in this spirit
the way will open for you to do more.
ROBERT COLLIER

WHAT KEEPS YOU so frozen in time that you can't find the energy or wherewithal to break loose and be who you are now? Is it an old tape playing back something belittling someone once said? Is it self-judgment, doubt, and criticism? Is it a fear of change?

Those questions always cycle in my head whenever I'm challenged to prove to myself that I'm not the hopeless klutz my father said I was. Ridding myself of his messages has been a difficult task. Consciously, I do my best to ignore them. But, I've learned, every once in a while they still sneak in the back door of my mind and blindside me. Like yesterday.

After a hearty breakfast at our vacation home, Ted, our friends Dan and Lisby, and I set out on our cross-country skis. Years earlier, I had tried skiing and actually got some momentum going. But too much time had passed, and as the three of them glided effortlessly into the woods, I began plodding—one slow, gooselike step after another.

For them, the day became a wonderful excursion interspersed with episodes of hurrying up and waiting. Hurry down the wooded hills to enjoy the thrill of the ride; wait for Caren to catch up, pick herself up, and figure out her next move. Frustrated, I kept pleading, "Don't wait for me. Just keep going."

With each stop, I felt as frozen as everything around me. Familiar tears and deep feelings of inadequacy kept surfacing. "You can go forward or you can go back," I finally told myself. "Which will it be?"

The vow "No going back, no going back" became my mantra as I struggled to catch up again. This time I found them looking down a long, steep hill. First Lisby went—crash. Then Dan—crash. Then Ted—crash. Then me. One calculated step at a time toward my destination. One step and another and another and a few tears and some sniffles and no crash and at the end a crooked smile and the joy of liberation.

■

AFFIRMATION

Whenever I become conscious of ties that bind me to the past,

I begin to set myself free.

■

No one is free who does not lord over himself.
Claudius

The secret of happiness is freedom,
and the secret of freedom is courage.
Thucydides

LIFE

the physical, mental, and spiritual experiences
that constitute existence; the interval of time
between birth and death

■

Even when I'm sick and depressed, I love life.
ARTHUR RUBENSTEIN

Life is what happens when you're making other plans.
JOHN LENNON

Life is raw material. We are artisans. We can sculpt our existence into
something beautiful, or debase it into ugliness. It's in our hands.
CATHY BETTER

EVERY TIME I attend or facilitate a workshop on self-healing, I keep a journal. Invariably, when I reread one of them, I usually discover that somewhere—in the gutters, in the margins, or along the tops of pages, as well as in bodies of text—I've jotted down the words "Choose life." This edict, which is attributed to the almighty God of the Jewish people, is in the book of Deuteronomy. "I call heaven and earth to witness against you today that I have set before you life and death, blessings and curses," proclaims the Divine. "Choose life so that you and your descendents may live."

Several times when I've written those powerful words, images of my children come to mind. They do now, and in this moment, I see tears of grief trickling down their faces on the night their father and I told them we were getting a divorce.

"I know how badly it hurts," I remember saying all those years ago to nine-year-old Jamie and six-year-old Evan. "We both love you so much and it feels so bad to have to tell you this," I added, all too aware of how inadequate my words sounded.

Like every couple repeating marriage vows, John and I believed that only death could separate us. In the years that followed, I learned that death wears many guises.

Our marriage died slowly, because we kept struggling to keep it alive. However, no matter how hard I tried, I felt the relationship becoming more life-draining than life-giving. John's alcoholism affected everyone in our family, as did my enabling and codependent behaviors.

One evening, after years of feeling as though the part of me that once loved John had died, I looked at Jamie and Evan playing joyfully together. Then I looked at John reading a book with one hand and holding his sixth beer of the evening in the other. And in that instant I knew what it meant to "Choose life," so that my descendents and I might live.

■

AFFIRMATION

Today, when look at what's set before me, I will choose life!

■

**He who postpones the hour of living is like the rustic who waits
for the river to run out before he crosses.**
HORACE

**When you were born, you cried and the world rejoiced.
Live your life so that when you die, the world cries and you rejoice.**
CHEROKEE PROVERB

LISTEN

to make an effort to hear something;
to pay attention

■

The fear of being alone with ourselves is . . . a feeling of
embarrassment, bordering sometimes on terror at seeing a person at
once so well known and so strange; we are afraid and run away. We
thus miss the chance of listening to ourselves,
and we continue to ignore our conscience.
ERICH FROMM

The soul is audible, not visible.
HENRY WADSWORTH LONGFELLOW

Learning to listen to ourselves is a way of learning to love ourselves.
JOAN BORYSENKO

ABOUT TEN YEARS ago, a late night call awakened us. "I think Tom may be dead," a neighbor told Ted. "I haven't seen him for several days and mail is piling up on his porch. I've called the police, but knew I should call you, too."

Immediately, we headed over to Tom's house. Two policemen wearing plastic gloves met us at the door. "He had AIDS and committed suicide, so you can't go in there or touch him," one said.

"I'm his minister," Ted replied. "I'm going to say prayers for him."

As Ted started in, a policeman blocking his entry said, "I don't think you heard me. He had A-I-D-S."

"Listen," Ted demanded. "I'm his minister and I'm going in to say prayers."

When the policemen finally backed away, we found Tom, thirty-one, spread out on the floor and clutching the bottle of pills he had swallowed. His note said he could no longer bear the endless pain, depression, and uncertainty caused by his intractable disease. Ted kneeled next to Tom's lifeless body, placed a hand on his shoulder, and began praying. Within moments, Tom's elderly, estranged mother arrived. Again the police blocked the entryway.

"But this is my son," she said, frantically. "I must see him." They refused. This time she begged. Finally, after listening to her pleadings, the police let her enter.

"Put these on," they said while handing her plastic gloves. She refused the gloves and sat down on the floor beside her son.

As Tom's mother gently wiped his matted hair away from his closed eyes, her tears wet his cheeks. After removing the empty bottle from his hand, she placed her arms around him. We listened as she expressed her sorrow, confusion, anger, and pain over Tom's choice to take his life. And then, as she rocked her baby boy in his eternal sleep, we heard her whisper words that she must have hoped Tom could still hear—heartfelt, healing words of love, forgiveness, and gratitude that he had been her son.

AFFIRMATION

When I listen to my heart, I hear healing words.

**The reason why we have two ears and only one mouth
is that we may listen the more and talk the less.**
ZENO OF CITIUM

He listens to good purpose who takes note.
ITALIAN PROVERB

LOVE

a strong predilection or enthusiasm; an intense emotional attachment

■

Love cures people—both the ones who give it
and the ones who receive it.
KARL MENNINGER

[Love] is not something that we must create, it *is* us. Love is our
essence—the fundamental energy that nourishes us. It is our birthright.
BENJAMIN SHIELD

The common denominator of all healing methods
is unconditional love—a love that respects the uniqueness of each individual and empowers each person to take responsibility
for his or her own well-being.
JACK SCHWARTZ

FROM THE TIME I was a child, the Jewish prayer called the Shema has always been both a comfort and a challenge to me. A comfort, because both the ancient words and the chant that accompanies them are in my blood and bones. A challenge, because every time I read the words "You shall love the LORD your God with all your heart, and with all your soul, and with all your might," I wonder what this commandment is really asking me to do.

What does it mean to be in a relationship and love with *all* of my heart, all of my soul, and all of my might? The job of loving a Divine being or others or myself with just the perfect, pretty, practical, positive parts of my body, psyche, and soul feels difficult enough. But if I am to love with *all,* does it mean that I have to factor into the process all those parts of me that I despise, detest, deny, and doubt, too?

Variations of the Shema appear several times in Judeo-Christian texts. In the Gospel stories, the text includes loving "with all your strength, and with all your mind; and your neighbor as yourself," Do this, Jesus tells a lawyer, and you will live.

Again I'm challenged. What does it mean to love my neighbor as myself? Whom do I usually love first? And why must I love with *all* to have life? When I look at the combined list—heart, soul, strength, mind, might, self (which can also mean one's resources)—I can't see any part of me that's excluded. Yet I know there are fractured, fragmented, and forsaken parts that I have yet to bring to consciousness. Must I be aware of *all* of them before I can love? Or do I get to know and include them because I love with all that I am here and now?

■

AFFIRMATION

The measure of love I give to myself and others
determines the life I get in return.

■

One word frees us of all the weight and pain of life; that word is love.
SOPHOCLES

Love can make any place agreeable.
ARABIAN PROVERB

MAPS

*a representation, usually on a
plane surface, of a region*

■

There is a great deal of unmapped country within us
which would have to be taken into account in an explanation
of our gusts and storms.
GEORGE ELIOT

I have an existential map; it has you are here written all over it.
STEPHEN WRIGHT

If you don't know where you are going,
how can you expect to get there?
BASIL S. WALSH

I'M SURE YOU'VE never heard of my cousin Abraham Zacuto. Yet we all owe him some gratitude. Cousin "Abe," who lived in the fifteenth century, was the court astronomer to two Spanish kings. His copper astrolabe enabled sailors to determine the position of the sun with greater precision; his improved astronomical tables permitted them to calculate latitudes and determine solar and lunar eclipses with greater accuracy. One ship's captain in particular depended upon my cousin's maps. His name was Christopher Columbus. Today, records with Columbus's annotations show that more than once Zacuto's calculations saved him from certain death while at sea and amongst hostile natives in Jamaica. Centuries later, cartography tools have changed. However, our dependence upon maps to give us direction and, possibly, save our lives remains the same.

Lying on a table in the oncology radiology department of Medical College of Ohio, I ponder the uncharted territories in my psyche and soul that I've visited since learning that a hostile, life-threatening disease named cancer had invaded my left breast. All the while, technicians are busy casting a topographical "map" of my northeast quadrant in styrofoam. It assures them that I'll always be properly aligned during my radiation treatments. I'm also there for my radiologist to literally map my chest with blue tattoos. When the needle pricks me, I flinch. A minute later three tiny blue dots rest inches apart on my breastbone. They look like Orion's belt. One more on my left side completes the permanent blueprint. "Will it ever be used again?" I wonder. "I hope not." But today, I'm glad they're there, because over the next six weeks, this map will guide the hands that will place and position me on the road to recovery.

Months later, I reach my destination. One morning as a mirror reflects my blue dots back to me, I express my gratitude for them. I'm at home and I'm safe and I'm well thanks to the maps that helped me to weather stormy waters and cross life-threatening terrain on my journey to health, healing, and wholeness.

■

AFFIRMATION

The maps I use on my healing journey guide me out of harm's way.

■

A traveller without knowledge is a bird without wings.
SA'DI

To be prepared is to have no anxiety.
KOREAN PROVERB

MEND

to improve in health or condition; to make
repairs or corrections

■

[In the Orient people believed] that the basis of all disease
was unhappiness. Thus to make a patient happy again
was to restore him to health.
DONALD LAW

Mending is a good metaphor for daily spiritual life. . . .
We are valuable members of the human community when we take our
own moral inventory and make daily repairs for our mistakes.
MAVIS AND MERLE FOSSOM

We are such docile creatures, normally, that it takes a virus to jolt us
out of life's routine. A couple of days in a fever bed are, in a sense,
health-giving; the change in body temperature, the change in pulse
rate, and the change of scene have a restorative effect on the
system equal to the hell they raise.
E.B. WHITE

NOT LONG AGO, I took a workshop to learn how to build stone walls. In silence, I began at one end and spent three days silently fitting, chiseling, and seaming stones together. Upon finally reaching the center of my side of the wall, I looked up at the name tag worn by a man who had just reached the same place on the opposite side. Noting not his name, but that he was from the same town where Ted once served a congregation before we met, I broke my silence.

"Small world," he said awkwardly when we established that he had been one of Ted's parishioners. At first, I thought it strange that upon closing our six degrees of separation he looked so uncomfortable. Then, as I gazed at his name for the first time I suddenly knew why. Before me stood the father of a reckless driver who had hit a tree at seventy miles per hour seventeen years earlier. My stepson, Chris, who was thirteen years old and a front-seat passenger, suffered major head injuries in the crash. This man's son walked away uninjured, and he was never prosecuted. Today, Chris's primary mode of transportation is his wheelchair.

Throughout our marriage, I have shared Ted's and Chris's pain over that accident. And although scars cover the physical and psychic wounds it caused, on rare occasions this protective mortar cracks. That day last summer, as I looked into the eyes of a stranger who now was no stranger at all, I felt vulnerable. Yet, intuitively, I knew what I had to do. I extended my hand over *our* wall. Tentatively, he extended his hand, too. And then, in silence, we each returned to our own work.

■

AFFIRMATION

Whenever I tie loose threads together, I help to mend the fabric of my life.

■

It is better to repair the beginning than the end.
GERMAN PROVERB

He who does not repair a gutter has a whole house to repair.
SPANISH PROVERB

MORNING

the first or early part; the dawn

■

There is a moment in the dawn . . .
when we see all things more truly than at any other time.
HENRY DAVID THOREAU

For what human ill does not dawn seem to be an alternative?
THORNTON WILDER

Every morning I wake up saying, I'm still alive; a miracle.
And so I keep on pushing.
JACQUES-YVES COUSTEAU

THIS MORNING, LIKE every morning, I said "Yes!" when I awakened. Today I whispered the word, but sometimes I just mouth it. Sometimes I say it out loud, and sometimes I just listen to the voice inside my head making it a mantra. Today and every day, it's the way I choose to affirm my return to conscious life and light from the land of my dreams and darkness.

Recently, Ted and I decided to downsize our living quarters. For ten years we have lived as urban pioneers in a large hundred-year-old Victorian home in a diverse inner-city neighborhood considered dangerous by outsiders. Their fears are not unwarranted. Some nights you can hear the "pop, pop, pop" of a gun being fired. The sound of sirens breaking the nighttime silence is common. Twice we awakened at night to the noise vandals made as they smashed the windshield on our car. Once we discovered the window in our garage had vanished overnight, along with our new bicycles. The unwritten law of the land in our old neighborhood is that you don't walk alone at night.

But morning is different. In Toledo's Old West End, morning has its own way of breaking the law. At dawn, people there, as everywhere, take to the streets with their routines. However, their waves, nods, and "Good morning" exchanges feel friendlier. Lots of children—always a sign of new life—head for school, and as you and the stranger coming your way look in each other's eyes, there's a feeling that a gap is being bridged, a wound is healing.

For me, the morning is the most healing time of the day. Today, at 5:00 A.M., as I look out my office window, a full moon stares back at me. In the silence, I hear myself philosophize over my many musings. These morning thoughts are unexpected visitors, said the Sufi poet Rumi. So I follow his advice and treat them honorably, because in this early hour, I'm not aware of what they may already know about this day. All I know is that right now they connect the darkness that's fading with the light that is dawning. This morning I feel new life. "Yes!"

■

AFFIRMATION

Today I will treat everything the morning brings like a guest in my house.

■

The morning hour has gold in its mouth.
GERMAN PROVERB

A misty morning does not signify a cloudy day.
PROVERB

MUSIC

*the art of arranging sounds in time
so as to produce a continuous, unified,
and evocative composition, as through melody,
harmony, rhythm, and timbre*

■

What we play is life.
LOUIS ARMSTRONG

**Music was my refuge. I could crawl into the spaces betwen the notes
and curl my back to loneliness.**
MAYA ANGELOU

**Every disease is a musical problem. Its cure a musical solution.
The more rapid and complete the solution,
the greater the musical talent of the doctor."**
NOVALIS

M Y DEAR FRIEND Deforia Lane, Ph.D., pioneered the use of music
therapy in hospitals nationwide. Although at one time Deforia aspired
to be an opera singer, after surviving two bouts of breast cancer she felt
called to become a music therapist instead. Today, almost twenty years later,
as the healthcare professionals at Ireland Cancer Center in Cleveland, Ohio,
treat the bodies of people with chronic and life-threatening diseases,
Deforia tends to their souls. The following story is about one of Deforia's
first patients, a teenager named Ginny.

"She was bandaged from head to foot and looked every bit like a
mummy. Only her eyes, mouth, and three fingers on her right hand
remained visible," recalls Deforia. "Complications in Ginny's leukemia
treatments had caused both her skin and beautiful red hair to fall off. Her

pain, similar to that of a burn patient, was unimaginable. She could only see shadows and was withdrawn and severely depressed."

Before visiting Ginny for the first time, Deforia learned that the teenager had a real flair for music. As she tentatively entered the room, Deforia said, "I've brought this strumming instrument with me. For you, playing it will be a piece of cake. It's called an Omnichord and you may play it today or I could come back another time." While waiting for Ginny to make a choice, Deforia softly strummed the autoharp-like instrument. Finally, Ginny declared, "I'll play now."

For the next forty-five minutes, Ginny sang and played her heart out with her three unbandaged fingers. All the while her mother and aunt cried. At one point, Deforia joined in and sang the popular song "That's What Friends Are For" to Ginny. "On the way out," Deforia said, "her mother told me that was the first time her daughter had smiled since she entered the hospital."

That was Friday, and over the weekend, Ginny, seventeen, died. Deforia attended her memorial service and, at Ginny's mother's request, once again offered the healing gift of music:

> Keep shining, keep smiling. . . .
> I'll be on your side forevermore.
> That's what friends are for.

■

AFFIRMATION

The sounds of music heal and harmonize my body, mind, and soul.

■

Music and rhythm find their way into the secret places of the soul.
PLATO

Music is the medicine of a troubled mind.
LATIN PROVERB

MYSTERY

*something not understood
or beyond understanding*

■

Who in the world am I? Ah, that's the great puzzle.
LEWIS CARROLL

The greatest mystery is in unsheathed reality itself.
EUDORA WELTY

Man can learn nothing except by going from
the known to the unknown.
CLAUDE BERNARD

FOR YEARS, MY daughter, Jamie, and I were estranged from each other. Whenever we would attempt to reconcile our differences, Jamie would do something to betray a trust that Ted and I placed in her. Each time that happened, the rift between us grew wider and wider. Eventually, Jamie distanced herself so much that we didn't know where to find her.

The pain of our fractured relationship hurt deeply. I was rooted in a family in which it was common for relatives on both sides to disown parents, children, and siblings and treat them as though they were dead. Now, despite promises to myself that I would not allow history to repeat itself, I was watching it happen. I vowed our door would always be open so Jamie could walk in anytime she felt ready to.

Three silent years passed before Ted and I learned from a friend that Jamie was in Key West, Florida, and doing well. I prayed for the right opportunity for me to knock on her door or for her to knock on ours.

One afternoon, the phone rang. I picked up and said hello. "Mom?" said a voice on the other end. The sound of traffic in the background suggested the caller was on a pay phone in a busy public place. "Jamie? Jamie? Is that you?" I asked.

"Yes, mom, it's me. I'm coming home, mom. I'm coming home." Before I could say another word, our phones disconnected.

"Jamie. Jamie?" Nothing. Stunned, I turned to Ted.

We waited for Jamie to call back, but she didn't. The next day, I located her phone number and nervously dialed it. "Jamie?" I said to the voice who picked up on the first ring.

"Mom?" she replied. "Mom?"

"Jamie, did you call me yesterday?"

"No. I didn't," she answered. For many moments, we were both silent. Finally, Jamie spoke. "Mom, can you forgive me?" she asked. "I want to come home."

■

AFFIRMATION

Today I will look for the healing that may lie
hidden in my unsolved mysteries.

■

You have hidden the truth in darkness;
through this mystery you teach me wisdom.
PSALMS 51:6

A riddle made by God is not solved.
AFRICAN PROVERB

NATURE

*the essential characteristics and qualities
of a person or thing; primitive state of
existence, untouched and uninfluenced
by civilization or artificiality*

■

Nature balances mind, body, and spirit
as co-creators of our personal reality.
DEEPAK CHOPRA

The art of medicine consists in amusing the patient
while nature cures the disease.
VOLTAIRE

I believe in God, only I spell it Nature.
FRANK LLOYD WRIGHT

EIGHT WEEKS AFTER I finished radiation treatments to destroy any renegade cancer cells still lurking in my breast, Ted and I began a scheduled
sabbatical. We spent most of it at Berkana. Whenever we're there, it seems
that Mother Nature always gifts us with something we haven't noticed
before. One morning, we awakened to see an entire flock of bright yellow
grosbeaks land on our deck railing. Another time, a bear paraded her two
cubs across that same stage.

Usually, these unexpected visitations give me pause to reflect upon the
vast natural world rather than my everyday parochial interests. So it was on
sabbatical that, for the first time, I noticed the numerous fungi growing on
the ground, on the trees, and even on some rocks. Large, small, hard, soft,
and coral-like protuberances colored yellow, orange, white, gray, red, blue,

brown, and even purple would seem to appear magically out of nowhere. Curiously, as each new discovery arrested my attention, it also reminded me that just months earlier my surgeon had dug an ugly, intrusive, funguslike growth out of my chest. It, too, had seemed to appear spontaneously.

To me, the internal fungus I had harbored was an alien invader bent upon destroying my inner world. At Berkana, I was discovering colorful by-products of decay in the outer world that provide healthful food for people, deer, and other animals and that also shelter toads, insects, and, says my granddaughter, fairies.

Why had I never paid attention to the fungi growing on and around other life-forms at Berkana before? What might the outer world be trying to tell me about the nature of my inner world and my healing process? For me, both the fungus I had felt hidden within my breast and the fungi I found in plain sight were wake-up calls from Mother Nature telling me to look around and see that the nature of healing is not about an either/or but a both/and process.

■

AFFIRMATION

What I see in the natural world around me reflects my true nature.

■

Nature, time, and patience are the three great physicians.
BULGARIAN PROVERB

Natural forces are the healers of disease.
HIPPOCRATES

NOURISH

to provide with food or other substances
necessary for life and growth;
to foster the development of

■

Whatever plows the body turns to food.
MURIEL RUKEYSER

Whenever you are sincerely pleased you are nourished.
RALPH WALDO EMERSON

The choice is between attacking and nourishing. You can see your body
as an enemy that has to be conquered, or you can consider it a friend
that needs to be cared for and supported so that health and well-being
will flourish. As sages the world over have affirmed for centuries, love
is the greatest healer there is.
MIRKA KNASTER

LIKE MANY PEOPLE who suffer from eating disorders and substance
abuse, my mother never realized how malnourished she looked. Several
times, her efforts to please my father's demands that she be perfect and have
a pencil-thin body on which he could hang beautiful clothes and exquisite
jewelry almost cost her her life. Indeed, today I still viscerally remember
times when, out of sheer frustration and despair, Mom attempted suicide
and I watched her life-nourishing blood literally going down the drain.

After twenty-five years of feeling starved for a healthy relationship to herself and her daughters, my mother finally left my father. The divorce that followed was bitter. For years afterwards, my mother continued to abuse herself, until one day she scrutinized her image in the mirror as though she were
looking through a new lens at the skeleton-like stranger she had become. "It

was so frightening," she told me. "I saw this horrible-looking woman and knew she was not just a reflection of my body, but my mind and soul, too."

Over the next ten years, my mother self-healed her body, mind, and spirit. She finally attained a healthy weight, quit drinking and smoking, and reconnected with her long-forgotten religious tradition. "I haven't felt this safe, secure, or nourished since my grandmother cradled me in her arms," she said during a visit.

Author M.F.K. Fisher once wrote, "It seems to me that our three basic needs for food and security and love, are so mixed and mingled and entwined that we cannot straightly think of one without the others." With that, my mother agreed.

◾

AFFIRMATION

I affirm my intention to nourish my body, mind, and spirit with self-love.

◾

If you ask a hungry man how much is two and two,
he replies four loaves.
HINDU PROVERB

At feasts, remember that you are entertaining two guests:
body and soul. What you give to the body, you presently lose,
what you give to the soul, you keep forever.
EPICTETUS

Now!

the present time or moment

■

The only way to live is to accept each minute as an unrepeatable miracle, which is exactly what it is: a miracle and unrepeatable.
STORM JAMESON

You don't get to choose how you're going to die. Or when.
You can only decide how you're going to live now.
JOAN BAEZ

I can feel guilty about the past, apprehensive about the future,
but only in the present can I act. The ability to be in the present
moment is a major component of mental wellness.
ABRAHAM MASLOW

IN 1997, AUTHOR Ram Dass, who through his works and good deeds is
considered a sage, suffered a major stroke. A year later, he was able to
talk, but he spoke haltingly and still groped for words. At a large benefit for
Ram Dass's medical care, friends gathered to hear him speak. After noting
that he felt it was tacky to come to one's own benefit and that's why he
came, Ram Dass addressed his predicament and the question of identity:

> For years I practiced as a karma yogi, the path of service. I wrote books
> about learning to serve, about how to help others. Now it is reversed. I need
> people to help me get up and put me to bed. Others feed me and wash my
> bottom. And I can tell you it's harder to be the one who is helped than the
> helper!
>
> But this is just another stage. It feels like I died and have been reborn over
> and over. In the sixties I was a professor at Harvard, and when that ended I
> went out with Tim Leary spreading LSD. Then in the seventies I died from that

and returned from India as Baba Ram Dass, the guru. Then in the eighties my life was all about service—cofounding the Seva Foundation, building hospitals, and working with refugees and prisoners. Over all these years I played cello, golf, drove my MG. Since this stroke the car is in the driveway, the cello and golf clubs in the closet. Now if I think I'm the guy who can't play cello or drive or work in India, I would feel terribly sorry for myself. But I'm not him. During the stroke I died again, and now I have a new life in a disabled body. This is where I am. You've got to be here now. You've got to take the curriculum.

■

AFFIRMATION

When I am aware of where I am now,
I see each moment as an unrepeatable miracle.

■

There is only one time when it is essential to awaken.
That time is now.
THE BUDDHA

If not now, when?
TALMUD

OBSTACLE

something that prevents action
or slows progress

■

Pursue the obstacle. It will set you free.
MARK NEPO

Mountain! Get out of my way!
MONTEL WILLIAMS

If you find a path with no obstacles,
it probably does not lead anywhere.
FRANK A. CLARK

A KING HAD A boulder placed on a roadway, hid himself, and watched to see if anyone would remove it. Some of the wealthiest merchants and courtiers in the realm came by and simply walked around it. Many loudly blamed the king for not keeping the roads clear, but did nothing about getting the big stone out of the way. Then a peasant came along carrying a load of vegetables. On approaching the boulder, he laid down his burden and tried to move the stone to the side of the road. After much pushing and straining, he finally succeeded. As the peasant picked up his load of vegetables, he noticed a purse lying in the road where the boulder had been. It contained many gold coins and a note from the king indicating that the gold was for the person who removed the boulder from the roadway.

My stepson Chris knows a lot about obstacles. Ever since he suffered severe head injuries in a car accident, Chris's constant companion is his wheelchair. When you're with him, it's difficult not to think about obstacles. Wheelchairs don't fit through standard doorways. Bathrooms aren't necessarily on the first floor. People don't always have patience when your cognitive problems keep you from finding words to express yourself.

Yet, despite boulder-sized stumbling blocks, I've watched Chris make stepping stones of many of them. Some, like having to travel rocky and rutted roads, require persistence and patience. Others, such as inaccessible bathrooms, require the courage and self-confidence needed to ask others for help. And not having words requires imagination and creativity, so that one can paint a picture of one's needs in other ways.

Over the last seventeen years, Chris has become adept at removing obstacles on his path to healing and wholeness. When he succeeds, his contagious smile indicates that he's found a purse of gold. Each time he makes me more cognizant of my physical limitations. He also makes me wonder, what obstacles do I have to persistently, courageously, confidently, patiently, and creatively work at removing to discover the hidden gold in my psyche and soul?

■

AFFIRMATION

Today I will choose to see the obstacles on my healing path
as stepping stones instead of stumbling blocks.

■

The obstacle is the path.
CHINESE PROVERB

**He who is outside his door already has the
hard part of the journey behind him.**
DUTCH PROVERB

OPPOSITES

altogether different, as in nature,
quality, or significance

■

Doublethink means the power of holding two contradictory beliefs in
one's mind simultaneously, and accepting both of them.
GEORGE ORWELL

It is the stretched soul that makes music, and souls are stretched by the
pull of opposites . . . where energies flow smoothly in one
direction—there will be much doing but no music.
ERIC HOFFER

Our existence seesaws between animality and divinity, between that
which is more and that which is less than humanity.
ABRAHAM JOSHUA HESCHEL

WHERE ARE THE places in your life where the light and the dark inter-
mingle, where the potential for embracing paradox and incongruity
intersect, where either/or can become a both/and, where life as you know
it can move outside the box?

Ted remembers such a time before and during his divorce when he and his
former spouse felt deeply wounded by each other and great sadness over their
loss. To his surprise, as many of the technical details fell quickly into place, a
battle began to rage over who would get certain possessions. "On the one
hand, I just wanted to give up everything and be finished. On the other, I
wanted what I felt was mine after twenty-three years of marriage," he recalls.

No one could come up with a solution, he explained, until one day, "as a
friend and I drove two hours to a meeting, I began telling him all about a
sideboard that was in my family for generations. When I finished the story,

something shifted. I felt as though I no longer had to hang onto it. So I opened the car window and symbolically let Granny's cabinet fly away. I then told stories about everything else I had hoped to keep and how my former wife and I came to possess those items. At the end of each story, I opened the window and let it go. By the time we got to the meeting, I felt different. I knew that my memories of what was good about my marriage were my real possessions and that I could live out of abundance, not scarcity. Whatever I actually got would be more than enough."

"Magic is present in those sacred spaces where opposites touch," says Kat Duff, author of *The Alchemy of Illness*. "Miracles of healing can occur at these intersections, although they are not necessary or inevitable, but simply demonstrations of grace."

■

AFFIRMATION

I invite healing possibilities into my life
when I live in the tension of opposing desires.

■

The excessive increase of anything causes a reaction
in the opposite direction.
PLATO

I call heaven and earth to witness against you today that I have set
before you life and death, blessings and curses.
DEUTERONOMY 30:19

OPTIMISM

a tendency to expect the best possible outcome

■

The optimist already sees the scar over the wound;
the pessimist still sees the wound underneath the scar.
ERNEST SCHRODER

Optimism is the cheerful frame of mind that enables a
teakettle to sing, though in hot water up to its nose.
HAROLD HELFER

The essence of optimism is that it . . . enables a man to hold his head
high, to claim the future for himself and not abandon it to his enemy.
DIETRICH BONHOFFER

RABBI MENACHEM MENDEL SCHNEERSON, who headed the Jewish Lubavitcher movement for forty-four years before his death in 1994, was known simply as "the Rebbe." Respected worldwide as a sage and a visionary, the Rebbe viewed health holistically. "Good health is far more than having a temperature of 98.6 degrees. Good health is a sound soul in a sound body," he wrote.

Moreover, "optimism, reinforced by a trust in G-d,* is just as important to the healing process as medicine and doctors."

According to a story told by Rabbi Simon Jacobson, who compiled the Rebbe's writings into a book, *Toward a Meaningful Life: The Wisdom of the Rebbe*, the Rebbe suffered a serious heart attack in 1977. The next day, he still insisted upon giving a talk to his following, just as he had for the previous thirty-eight years. A few days later, when a doctor asked the Rebbe how he was feeling, he said, "Physically, thank G-d, I feel fine. But mentally, I'm not so well." This, the Rebbe went on to tell the doctor, was probably due to the fact that he had not been able to spend time in silent prayer and contemplation at the graveside of his beloved father-in-law and predecessor. Normally, he did this several times a month.

"You must take care of your health," the doctor insisted. "If not, there is a twenty-five percent chance of a relapse." The doctor then asked if the Rebbe understood what he had said.

"Oh yes," replied the Rebbe with a smile. "You said that even if I don't take care of my health—which, I assure you, I will—there is a seventy-five percent chance that there won't be a relapse."

Another time, when a hospital administrator came to the Rebbe for a blessing, he told the Rebbe that he worked in a "house of the sick." The Rebbe then suggested his visitor might call it a "house of doctors" or "house of healing" instead. The difference, the Rebbe explained, is that when a patient enters a hospital and feels that he is entering a house of healing instead of a house of sickness, it lifts his morale and encourages the healing process.

■

AFFIRMATION

Today I will try to see every half-empty glass as half-full.

■

Whatever is, is right.
GREEK PROVERB

Keep on sowing your seed, for you never know which will grow—
perhaps it all will.
ECCLESIASTES 11:6

*Out of respect for the Third Commandment, "You shall not take the Lord your God's name in vain," it is common for Jewish people to spell God G-d or G-D.

PASSION

intense, driving, or overmastering
feeling or conviction

■

Between the two pressures of passion and identity we create a life.
THOMAS MOORE

Being on the tightrope is living; everything else is waiting.
KARL WALLENDA

**Whenever people are totally caught up . . . in their passion—a timeless
quality exists in which they are expressing the real essence of their
authentic self. And this genuine essence, this authentic self, thereby
helps their inner love grow.**
JEAN SHINODA BOLEN

AUTHOR AND PHILOSOPHER Sam Keen is passionate about flying, but not
airplanes, kites, or hot air balloons. For Keen, flying equates with the
word *trapeze*—trapeze as in the circus. And ever since shortly after his sixty-
second birthday, when he saw an ad offering instruction on how to fly on a
trapeze, he's been floating on air.

In his book *Learning to Fly*, Keen reminisces about his childhood dream of
flying and admits that the qualms that surfaced when finally faced with the
possibility were generated by his fear that he might now be too old. But
despite all of his concerns, an animating life force that Keen calls "passion"
ruled.

"Passion is seldom rational and usually blind," he explains. "You can bet that
when you are suddenly swept away—abandon your marriage, take a new
lover, quit your job, buy a sailboat, run off with the circus—in due course you
will discover that the overt object of your affections is a surrogate for covert

longing that you hide even from yourself. Over the years I have discovered that it is hazardous to ignore passing fantasies and emerging passions."

The root of the word *passion* is in the Latin *pati*—"suffer." If we ignore our deepest passions, we will suffer, because our deepest fears seize that opportunity to move into the driver's seat. "When passion no longer waters and nurtures the psyche, fears spring up like weeds on the depleted soil of abandoned fields," observes Keen. In fact, he suspects that the major cause of the mood of depression and despair in our society may be rooted in the masses of people who are chained to jobs that do not engage their passion for creativity and meaning. Those who honor their passions, he concludes, rarely get stuck in who they are now. Instead, they begin to blossom into who they might be.

■

AFFIRMATION

When I honor my emerging passions, I begin blossoming into who I might be.

■

All human actions have one or more of these seven causes: chance, nature, compulsions, habit, reason, passion, desire.
ARISTOTLE

Passions are good servants and bad masters.
GREEK PROVERB

PEACE

the absence of war or other hostilities;
inner contentment; serenity

■

Looking for peace is like looking for a turtle with a mustache:
You won't be able to find it. But when your heart is ready,
peace will come looking for you.
AJAHN CHAH

I do not want the peace which passeth understanding.
I want the understanding which bringeth peace.
HELEN KELLER

Once we learn to touch peace, we will be healed and transformed. It is
not a matter of faith; it is a matter of practice.
THICH NHAT HANH

LAST CHRISTMAS, SOMEONE e-mailed me a true story about a peace that did, indeed, "pass all understanding." The event took place in Europe on Christmas day in 1914 during World War I. The night before, as darkness fell on the bloody battlefields, Sir Edward Hulse, a twenty-five-year-old lieutenant, journaled about a strange occurrence:

A scout named F. Marker went out and met a German Patrol and was given a glass of whisky and some cigars, and a message was sent back, saying that "if we didn't fire at them they would not fire at us." That night the fighting suddenly just stopped. The following morning, German soldiers walked toward the British lines while the British came out to greet their enemy. They exchanged souvenirs with each other and the British gave the German soldiers plum pudding as a Christmas greeting. Soon arrangements were made to bury the dead British soldiers whose bodies were lying in no man's land. The Germans brought the bodies over and prayers were exchanged. . . .

Another British soldier, Second Lieutenant Dougan Chater, also wrote about that Christmas in the trenches, when two Germans got out of theirs and headed toward his:

> We were just going to fire on them when we saw that they had no rifles so one of our men went out to meet them and in about two minutes the ground between the two lines of trenches was swarming with men and officers of both sides, shaking hands and wishing each other a happy Christmas. This continued for nearly an hour before their superiors ordered the men back.

Not long ago, a backstage cleaning woman told Grammy nominee John McCutcheon the WWI story. In response, he wrote a song about the peace that passed between the soldiers. The temporary truce wasn't an isolated incident, he says, but a series that spread along two-thirds of the disease-infested, muddy trenches on the Flanders fields of Belgium and France. How did McCutcheon know? Once, during a concert tour, three elderly German men traveled to Denmark to meet McCutcheon and "hear that song." They had been there.

■

AFFIRMATION

Let there be peace on earth, and let it begin with me.

■

May you have warmth in your igloo, oil in your lamp, and peace in your heart.
ESKIMO PROVERB

Inner peace is beyond victory or defeat.
BHAGAVAD GITA

PERSEVERANCE

steady persistence in adhering to a course of action, a belief, or a purpose

■

The best way out is always through.
ROBERT FROST

Persevering in one's existence is the particular quality of the organism;
it is not a progress toward achievement followed by stasis, which is the
machine's mode, but an interactive, rhythmic, and unstable process,
which constitutes an end in itself.
URSULA K. LEGUIN

I have become my own version of an optimist. If I can't make it through
one door, I'll go through another door—or I'll make a door. Something
terrific will come no matter how dark the present.
JOAN RIVERS

AFTER MY SURGEON removed a tiny malignant tumor from my left breast, he told me that I would need thirty-three radiation treatments to make sure any renegade cancer cells were destroyed. "Thirty-three!" I exclaimed anxiously to myself. "How will I ever withstand that much radiation? Why are they so sure it will help me instead of harm me? Isn't there something else I can do? What makes thirty-three so special instead of thirty-one or twelve?"

I told my surgeon I needed to think about it, talk to other women who had had radiation, get my other doctors' opinions, and do some reading. He supported my plan of action. Several days later, convinced I should undergo radiation, I called the hospital for my first appointment.

For five days a week over the next six and a half weeks, I underwent treatments to destroy something no one could see with something no one could see. Some days, as I looked at the massive equipment all around me, doubts filled empty places in my head and my heart. Weekends were my Sabbath—a time for my body and mind to rest and renew and reflect.

At first, this disruptive weekly routine seemed endless. But upon passing the halfway point, I suddenly felt that my perseverance was paying off. Time moved a little faster. My goal was in sight. It was then that I came across this quote by Jacob Riis, the American social reformer and writer. "When nothing seems to help," he wrote, "I go and look at a stonecutter hammering away at his rock perhaps a hundred times without as much as a crack showing in it. Yet at the hundred-and-first blow, it will split in two, and I know it was not that blow that did it, but all that had gone before." Such was the case, I believe, in steadfastly persevering in order to complete thirty-three radiation treatments—not one more, not one less.

■

AFFIRMATION

When I fortify my healing journey with perseverance,
I know every step—no matter how large or small—matters.

■

Pray to God, but keep rowing to shore.
RUSSIAN PROVERB

The man who removes a mountain begins by
carrying away small stones.
CHINESE PROVERB

PERSPECTIVE

*the relationship of aspects of a subject to each
other and to a whole; a view or vista*

■

Life can only be understood backwards;
but it must be lived forwards.
SØREN KIERKEGAARD

Tragedy and comedy are but two aspects of what is real, and whether
we see the tragic or the humorous is a matter of perspective.
ARNOLD BEISSER

Every man takes the limits of his own field of
vision for the limits of the world.
ARTHUR SCHOPENHAUER

AFTER THE CAR accident that permanently disabled Ted's son, Chris, the
people in his congregation would discount their misfortunes in light of
his. "I know this will seem insignificant compared to what's happened to
you," became a standard preface to any comments about their crises and
concerns. Ted, however, didn't see it that way.

"While Chris was still in the hospital, I got a call that the five-year-old
daughter of a parishioner was in the emergency room with a shattered arm,"
he said. "When I got there, distress and worry were written all over her parents' faces. She was sobbing uncontrollably because she was scared and in lots
of pain." According to Ted, they were a very religious family, and as they held
Katie and tried reassuring her that God and the doctors would make everything "all better," it was obvious that their failure to offer more consolation
or a miracle made them feel impotent. They also admitted feeling guilty that
they were unable to prevent the accident that had happened before their

eyes. "Yet, with all that was going on for them in those moments, they still said they hated to bother me. They kept saying, 'Ted, this is just a broken arm. It's nothing compared to what you're going through.' "

"We don't see things as they are, we see them as we are," said author Anaïs Nin. If we are truly to gain perspective when something shakes our foundations and turns our world upside down, we must carefully choose the lens through which we view our experience. Only then can we truly honor what *we* feel in our bodies, minds, and spirits and what, in their infinite wisdom, they might want us to know about *our* pain, suffering, and means of turning our world right side up.

"None of us can measure someone else's anguish or their resiliency," says Ted. "I saw Chris's accident from my perspective and everyone in my family saw it from theirs. Throughout that ordeal, I didn't hurt more and I didn't hurt less than anyone else, I just really hurt. And you know something? Seventeen years out there, every time I look back I still do—just not as much."

■

AFFIRMATION

*I will honor events in my life by seeing them in the
light of my perspective, not others'.*

■

**How much time he saves who does not look to see
what his neighbor says or thinks.**
MARCUS AURELIUS

Nothing's beautiful from every point of view.
HORACE

PLAY

*to occupy oneself in amusement, sport,
or other recreation; activity engaged in
for enjoyment or recreation*

■

We do not stop playing because we grow old;
we grow old because we stop playing.
ANON

When you're depressed, the whole body is depressed, and it translates to
the cellular level. The first objective is to get your energy up, and you can
do it through play. It's one of the most powerful ways of breaking up
hopelessness and bringing energy into the situation.
O. CARL SIMONTON

Play is the exultation of the possible.
MARTIN BUBER

O. FRED DONALDSON, PH.D. is a play specialist whose "work" includes playing with autistic children, street gang members, wolves, and grizzly bears. He believes that in early childhood we know, intuitively, that the game of life is there "to be *one*, not won." While discussing the healing power of free, noncompetitive play, Donaldson tells a story about a young man in his late thirties who was born with cerebral palsy:

We were in a ballroom when I asked Doug if he would like to get out of his wheelchair and play with me. He answered yes with so much enthusiasm that I thought he might leap out of the chair himself. After advising me how I could help him get out of his chair, we got down on the floor. There, like two boys on a lawn, we rolled around, tumbled over and under each other, and finally rested on the carpet—breathing heavily and hugging each other. Later, during dinner, Doug cried while telling me about his parents' fear of touching him. He explained that he had always wanted his father, who had recently died, to play with him. "But he never did," Doug said. "No one ever did."

Many years ago, I watched from the beach as my very young children played, gleefully, in Lake Erie with a friend of mine. All three kept urging me to join them. But whenever I tried to stand up, old messages shouting "No!" glued me to the sand. Suddenly, I realized for the first time that during most of my childhood my father had forbidden me to go outside and play. In turn, I had always found it difficult to frolic spontaneously with my children. "Never again," I shouted to the breaking waves. I then brushed away my tears and raced into the water to play with my children and the child in me.

■

AFFIRMATION

It's never too late to experience the healing power of play.

■

In our play we reveal what kind of people we are.
OVID

Life must be lived as play.
PLATO

PRAYER

*a specially worded form used to address and / or
petition God, a god,
or another object of worship*

■

Prayer does not change God, but it changes him who prays.
SØREN KIERKEGAARD

**Prayer is not an old woman's idle amusement. Properly understood and
applied, it is the most potent instrument of action.**
MAHATAMA GANDHI

To pray is to think about the meaning of life.
LUDWIG WITTGENSTEIN

EVEN THOUGH I don't have a clue how or why prayer works, I just know
that it does and that lots of evidence supports my belief. For example,
author and physician Larry Dossey has written about more than 130 con-
trolled laboratory studies that show, in general, that prayer or a prayerlike
state of compassion, empathy, and love can bring about healthful changes in
many types of living things, from humans to bacteria. "This does not mean
that prayer *always* works," he says, "any more than drugs and surgery always
work but that, statistically speaking, prayer is effective."

Although statistics bolster the claim for the efficacy of prayer, anyone
who has experienced its healing power knows that numbers are needed only
to convince skeptics. I was reminded of that last year, when my husband's
family gathered around my father-in-law's hospital bed to bid farewell to
this beloved man. A rare form of heart disease was exhausting Ed's life, and
we knew there were no other medical procedures or miracles to be pulled
out of his doctors' bags.

For hours before Ed's six children and their spouses arrived, my mother-in-law, Millie, had repeatedly wiped the brow, kissed the cheek, and embraced the fragile body of the semiconscious man with whom she had shared fifty-six years. Several times, when his breathing slowed so much it wouldn't float a feather, she expected him to die. But he lingered in a deepening coma instead.

However, it now seemed as though the time for Ed to pass had, at last, come. At first, we tried to make his transition more comfortable by singing "Amazing Grace." But we were a sorry lot that couldn't carry a tune, and Ed's agitated body language suggested we were possibly harming instead of healing. So we stopped and lapsed into silence. Minutes later, Ted began reciting The Lord's Prayer. Joining in, we held each other's hands. Millie gently squeezed one of Ed's and someone else his other. And as we slowly— ever so slowly—said the familiar words that Ed dearly loved, we also prayed that he could hear each one. He must have, because as we all sighed "Amen," he drew his last breath.

■

AFFIRMATION:

My prayers echo a still, small voice inside my body, mind, and soul.

■

**It is vain to expect our prayers to be heard
if we do not strive as well as pray.**
AESOP

A grateful thought toward heaven is a complete prayer.
GERMAN PROVERB

QUESTIONS

*an expression of inquiry or a point that invites
or calls for a reply or consideration*

■

Life is about not knowing, having to change, taking the moment
and making the best of it, without knowing
what's going to happen next. Delicious ambiguity.
GILDA RADNER

The only interesting answers are those which destroy the questions.
SUSAN SONTAG

The Serpent: You see things; and you say, "Why?"
But I dream things that never were; and I say, "Why not?"
GEORGE BERNARD SHAW

EVERY SUMMER, MY husband and I lead a nine-day seminar called "Living the Questions" at a retreat center in the Pocono Mountains. During the summer of 2000, I felt more like a student than a teacher. After undergoing treatment for cancer, losing my mother and father-in-law, and learning my daughter had multiple sclerosis—all within six months—I had spent lots of time asking myself: "Why? Why me? Why now? Why not? Where do I go from here? Why go anywhere?"

Like many people who experience the pain, disappointment, anxiety, and fear that accompany illness and death, I reasoned that the answers to those questions might mend the torn fabric of my life. However, my heart and soul knew better. Each time my head sought answers, words by the poet Rainer Maria Rilke would surface instead. "Be patient toward all that is unsolved in your heart and try to love the questions themselves," he said. "Do not now seek the answers which cannot be given you because you would not be able to live them. And the point is to live everything. *Live* the questions now. . . . "

So instead of seeking answers that summer, I spent a lot of time wondering: "What does it mean for me 'to *live* the questions?' What's required if I am to *love* the questions? What do questions do? What is the cost of asking questions? What might be the promise of asking questions? What's the appeal of answers? When am I most apt to want them? What's the cost of having answers? What about the promise? What's the cost of not having answers? The promise?"

Today, I still ponder those questions and others that they spawn. I know that it takes trust, faith, and courage to choose to have them accompany me on my healing path. That's why I try to see each as a stepping-stone leading me to the Tree of Life.

■

AFFIRMATION

Today I will have patience with all that is unsolved in my heart and try to love the unanswered questions that sit there.

■

Hard questions must have hard answers.
GREEK PROVERB

The question of a wise man is half the answer.
SOLOMON IBN GABIROL

REBIRTH

a second or new birth; a renaissance; a revival

■

Every day is a new life. Seize it. Live it.
DAVID GUY POWERS

New seed
is faithful.
It roots deepest
in the places
that are most empty.
CLARISSA PINKOLA ESTÉS

To live fully is to let go and die with each passing moment, and to be
reborn in each new one.
JACK KORNFIELD

ONE SUMMER, AT a seminar at a retreat center in northern California, our leader quoted Fritz Kunkel, a German psychiatrist: "Imagine yourself re-walking the path of your life when you come to a gravestone on which is inscribed, 'This is where I was first killed.' "

"Where's the place where you were first killed?" she then asked.

Flash! I see myself inside a hospital in 1947. Sam Markoff, our family doctor, smiles as he shows me to my father for the first time. "It's a beautiful girl," he says. But my father doesn't see it that way. He looks disappointed and turns his head away. I sense, immediately, that I am not acceptable. Before it all begins, a part of me dies.

The existential death that I believe I suffered on my birth day was the first of many I experienced every time my father said that he wanted me to be a boy. Desperate for some sign of recognition, seven-year-old I began reciting a special prayer at bedtime: "Please, please, please, God. Please, please, please let me be a boy when I wake up so Daddy will love me."

It didn't work. Nothing worked. Being a tomboy didn't help. I remained invisible. Morphing into a yin-and-yang teenager—wild on one hand and an honor student on the other—never got me acknowledgment. Neither did carving out a successful career as a writer. When at twenty I eloped with a Catholic, *that* arrested my father's attention—but only long enough for him to talk to his rabbi and then to say prayers for the dead in my name.

In spite of all those rejections, I continued to long to be acceptable in my father's sight. That is, until the day when a doctor in a delivery room placed the baby I had just brought into the world in my arms. And as they enfolded around the most beautiful girl I had ever seen, I looked right into her eyes and felt something new come alive deep inside of me. And for the first time ever, I felt profoundly grateful that I was a woman, and I thanked God that it was so.

■

AFFIRMATION

Awareness and insight awaken new life in me.

■

Behold! I am making all things new.
REVELATIONS 21:5

Do not be conformed to this world,
but be transformed by the renewal of your mind.
SAINT PAUL

REMEDY

something that relieves pain, cures disease,
or corrects a disorder

■

Every day, in every way, I am getting better and better.
ÉMILE COUÉ

Each person carries his own doctor within.
ALBERT SCHWEITZER

For every ailment under the sun,
There is a remedy,
or there is none.
If there be one,
try to find it;
If there be none,
never mind it.
MOTHER GOOSE

THE WORD *THROE* means a condition of agonizing struggle or trouble, and it is rooted in an Old English word for "pain and affliction." When organizations deep in the throes of conflict hire me to consult with them, their immediate hope is that I can provide them with a quick fix for their *dis*ease. "I wish I could," I tell them, "but I can't. Healing isn't about a topical remedy that you can slap on and cover up. Instead, healing is a process that takes time, patience, courage, and the ability to look at one's wounds from the inside out. I can't heal you. Only you can do that."

I then introduce the organization to a holistic healing process in which members begin to look at themselves as an organism—a whole interrelated system—and not just a group of individuals hanging out with each other.

The body, with its eyes, hands, heart, brain, ears, stomach, lungs, nerves, cells, and so on, is a good model. When each part functions as it should, it assures our health and contributes to our well-being and survival. However, if the nose continually runs, the stomach always feels unsettled, or a wound festers, it's a sign of dysfunction and possibly disease. Although cold medicine, an antacid, or a Band-Aid may mask the most superficial and obvious symptoms, it cannot heal the source of the discomfort and illness or jump start a faulty immune system. To get to the core of systemic problems and truly remedy them, all the contributing factors—inner and outer, past and present—must be exposed. Only then can the body's healthful responses be summoned into action.

Sadly, in an age of quick fixes for almost every problem, it can be hard to believe that even duct tape is only a temporary patch, not a permanent solution. Real remedies that can help heal our wounds can only be found when we are willing to take time, stay the course, and acknowledge how much our wounds hurt—not just physically, but emotionally and spiritually, too. Even then, we must face the possibility that while the remedy helped to heal us, we could not be cured.

■

AFFIRMATION

More and more I acknowledge that the gift of healing lies within me.

■

[Illness] bears its own remedy within itself. . . .
Health must grow from the same root as disease.
PARACELSUS

He who conceals his disease cannot expect to be cured.
ETHIOPIAN PROVERB

REMEMBER

*to recall to the mind; to return to (an original
shape or form) after being deformed or altered*

■

Some memories are realities and better than anything
that can ever happen to one again.
WILLA CATHER

As a life's work, I would remember everything—
everything against loss. I would go through life like a plankton net.
ANNIE DILLARD

All water has a perfect memory and is forever trying
to get back to where it was.
TONI MORRISON

For most of us, remembering means recalling memories. However,
when we *re-member* ourselves, we not only recall events that help us to
tie past to present, but we also engage in a healing process that reunites the
fragmented and disparate parts of our "selfs."

"When I think of events that rend the soul, my most pernicious image is
the Nazi Holocaust," says my friend Faye Sholiton. "It was the calculated
murder of millions of neighbors by neighbors. Most survivors suffered psychic and spiritual dismemberment and, until recently, rarely spoke about
their experiences. Now, however, as they enter their final decades, many are
summoning the courage to share their stories as a legacy to humankind."

Faye, an award-winning playwright and journalist, spent fifteen years
interviewing dozens of Holocaust survivors. In "The Interview," she drama-
tizes the twenty-four-hour period when Bracha Weissman, a feisty sixty-
nine-year-old death camp survivor, is preparing to tell her story to the

young woman who will take her testimony for an oral history project. Now widowed and alone, Bracha lives in a perfectly ordered world. When asked about the steps she took to rejoin the human race, Bracha replies, "You begin by learning how to use a fork and a toothbrush again. Then you jump into a marriage without ever having a courtship. Then you make love and babies and money and you go on—or make believe you do. . . ."

As the two women risk self-disclosure, Bracha soon discovers how profoundly her young interviewer, a child of survivors, was also affected by the same tragedy. And as she at last begins *re-membering* the wounded pieces of her shattered life, Bracha suddenly realizes she's helping another to do the same.

According to psychologist and author Elizabeth Boyden Howes, "There is somewhere deep in the heart of existence the most eternal struggle to heal the split between different parts of ourselves, between person and person, between the conscious and unconscious, between spirit and the substance, the light and dark, the up and the down. If we are aware of this and are committed to this process, we are working for the process that is God."

■

AFFIRMATION

When I summon the courage to call lost and forgotten parts of myself home,
I re-member my body, mind, and spirit.

■

How sweet to remember the trouble that is past!
GREEK PROVERB

Memory is the treasury and guardian of all things.
LATIN PROVERB

RESPONSIBILITY

the state, quality, or fact of being responsible

■

We are not responsible *for* our illnesses, we are responsible to them, to
what they offer and require of all of us, sick and well alike.
KAT DUFF

We are responsible for actions performed in response to circumstances for which we are not responsible.
ALLAN MASSIE

It is easier to do one's duty to others than to one's self. If you do your
duty to others, you are considered reliable. If you do your duty to yourself, you are considered selfish.
THOMAS SZASZ

MY FRIEND STEVEN ROSMAN, Ph.D., directs the complementary medicine department for one of the largest medical practices in New
York. Steve is also a rabbi, who enjoys telling this version of an old story:

Once it rained for days on end. When runoffs flooded the town, Mr.
Yetzer climbed to his roof for safety. However, the waters continued to rise
until they reached his roof and threatened to overwhelm him.

Just then a man came by in a rowboat. "Jump in!" cried the man. But Mr.
Yetzer said, "No, thanks. I am a man of faith and I am sure that the Lord will
save me."

Well, after that the waters continued to rise and reached to Mr. Yetzer's
ankles. Steadfastly, he continued to await his salvation—even when a helicopter hovered above him and dangled a rope-ladder in front of his nose.
"No, thanks," Mr. Yetzer said while waving away the helicopter crew. "I am a
man of faith, and I am sure that the Lord will save me."

The same thing happened when divers swam by. Mr. Yetzer refused their help and the lifesaver thrown his way. Finally, he drowned. In the world beyond, he faced his Master and wanted to know why Divine help had not saved him.

"Help came your way," was the response. "First I sent a rowboat, then a helicopter, then divers, and finally I sent you a lifesaver. You did not do your part."

Reflecting upon the story, Steve says that it's important to remain open to the fact that healing help may not come in expected ways. More than 1,500 years ago, the great Jewish rabbis advised their people not to rely on miracles. They taught that bread is not created in loaves; we have to mill and bake the wheat to make bread. Likewise, there's always a portion of responsibility each person must assume for his or her own welfare.

◼

AFFIRMATION

More and more I am willing to accept
a portion of responsibility for my well-being.

◼

A courtyard common to all will be swept by none.
CHINESE PROVERB

God gave burdens, also shoulders.
YIDDISH PROVERB

RISK

to expose to hazard or danger

◼

The fullness of life is in the hazards of life.
EDITH HAMILTON

And the day came when the risk to remain tight in a bud
was more painful than the risk it took to blossom.
ANAÏS NIN

Leap and the net will appear.
JULIA CAMERON

DAN AND LISBY POLLOCK know something of the wounds we may suffer when taking risks. Just a few years ago, when these good friends chose to sell their successful multimillion-dollar company to their employees, they knew there were inherent risks in their decision. So, to assure the future health of the company, their financial security, and a smooth transition, Dan personally groomed a longtime employee to be his successor, and he and Lisby met with some of the best consultants in the field. He also held mandatory meetings so that all of his employees would learn everything they needed to know about running their company and the changing of the guard.

The day Dan turned over the keys, both he and the company enjoyed peak health. However, just eleven months later, the company was on the verge of bankruptcy due to mismanagement and betrayals of his trust. Moreover, the bank threatened that Dan and Lisby could be personally liable for all of the company's debts.

"It was the most devastating, frightening thing that ever happened to me," Lisby said, months later. "We stood to lose everything. As the company died, so did a part of us. Finally, a buyer purchased the assets of the company. But our wounds continue to ache, and we still grieve the financial losses and emotional stress that so many good, honest people suffered."

Interestingly, when asked how he now feels about taking risks, Dan tells a story about a deceased friend named Jim, who always wanted to sail. Upon retiring, Jim bought the boat of his dreams so he could take it on the Chesapeake. Just days later, Jim's doctor told him that he had a very serious heart condition and that sailing might kill him. So he never did. Instead, Jim sold the boat and sat at home for twenty years before dying. "Selling the company turned out to be an adventure on high, stormy seas for me," says Dan. "The risk was greater than I ever envisioned. But you know something—I'd much rather die sailing."

■

AFFIRMATION

When I choose safety for safety's sake, I am not choosing life.

■

Biggest profits mean gravest risks.
CHINESE PROVERB

**It is not because things are difficult that we do not dare,
it is because we do not dare that they are difficult.**
SENECA

RITUAL

the established form for a ceremony;
a detailed method of procedure
faithfully or regularly followed

■

Ritual is routine infused with mindfulness. It is habit made holy.
KENT NERBURN

When rituals become ends in themselves it means we're stuck in their
form instead of flowing with their function.
TED VOORHEES

Rituals of healing have a profound sense of the sacred.
When we use them to renew the fabric of our lives that becomes unrav-
eled by change, chaos, illness, and death,
a sense of balance and harmony emerge that reconnect
our energies and meet our needs of the moment.
BARBARA DOSSEY

AT MY PARENTS' summer home in New Jersey, my father forged a very
strange relationship with his land. For reasons he refused to explain, he
would regularly order my sister, Deborah, or me to "pick rocks." Not just
one or a handful, but wheelbarrows full that we would push tearfully across
seven acres to a designated mound.

Not surprisingly, for years after freeing myself from that labor of
Sisyphus, I shied away from rocks. In college I never took a popular geolo-
gy course. In England I didn't visit Stonehenge. And during my first airplane
ride over the Rockies, I never looked down to see the majestic peaks below.
Not until I chose to climb a ninety-foot rock wall, to begin symbolically facing issues with my father, did a healing path appear.

Years later, as part of that healing journey, I began ritually unearthing rocks to line the sides of streams at our refuge in West Virginia. Today, I still do. Daily, my ritual includes heading out early in the day and wandering on our fifteen acres until one or more sandstone hunks call me to them. I then spend a couple of hours silently farming them with a shovel and a crowbar. My attention is undivided. Large stones can take days to unearth. Some must be rolled from their beds instead of lifted. Once finished for the day, I sit with my pickings, studying their contours and waiting, patiently, for them to reveal buried secrets about my relationship to others, our land, and myself.

In 1994, as my father lay dying, remnants of the huge rock pile my sister and I mounded still stood outside his bedroom window. Now covered in crabgrass and other weeds, it seemed like a snapshot of his hard, messy life. After his funeral, I wanted to ritually dismantle the pile stone by stone, but the thought of doing that offered me no hope. So, instead, I went to Berkana and walked to a favorite spot. And there, in my father's name, I unearthed and then blessed a new crop of stones.

■

AFFIRMATION

My healing rituals help me to repair the frayed fabric of my life.

■

There are hundreds of ways to kneel and kiss the ground.
RUMI

You have hidden the truth in darkness;
through this mystery you teach me wisdom.
PSALMS 51:6

SABBATH

a time of rest

■

The Sabbath rocks us and holds us
until we can remember who we are.
WAYNE MUELLER

Mentally, fallow is as important as seedtime.
Even bodies can be exhausted by overcultivation.
GEORGE BERNARD SHAW

When we work well, a Sabbath mood
Rests on our day, and finds it good.
WENDELL BERRY

For TED AND me, the word *Sabbath* usually means going to Berkana, our vacation home on densely wooded acreage in West Virginia. We dubbed our respite Berkana because we loved the sound and the sense of this Celtic word meaning "rebirth and renewal." From the beginning, we hoped it would be a place where we could spend and suspend time walking, talking, and sitting silently beside still waters that could restore our souls.

Each Sabbath at Berkana does renew our bodies and souls. However, it took a visit from my Jewish mother for me to appreciate fully the healing power of Shabbat, the holy day that she celebrated weekly.

In my mother's world, time stood still on Shabbat no matter where she was. That meant the first twenty-four hours of her first three-day visit to Berkana wouldn't be spent exploring breathtaking scenery by car or taking a midnight drive to a vast meadow to see the heavens through my telescope. It also meant we wouldn't be talking on the telephone to those elsewhere. Neither would we be cooking, writing, housecleaning, chopping wood, or carrying water. We would just be.

At first I worried, "What will we do?" Most of our lives we had been strangers to each other. In recent years we had repaired many of the rents in the fabric of our common lives, but on this visit, twenty-four hours seemed like a long time to unselfishly, wholeheartedly be—and just be—with my mother.

It wasn't long enough. At sundown, the beginning of Shabbat, we placed beautiful flowers in a vase, lit candles, and said traditional prayers. We ate the simple meal I had prepared earlier. And as we talked and talked and talked through the night and into the next day, she took me to places in her past that I had never known about. She introduced me to relatives I had never met. She revealed a sense of humor I had never appreciated. She spoke truths never before spoken, and she told me she loved me in ways I could never hear before.

My mother died before I could gift her with another visit to Berkana. At Berkana, my mother gifted me with something everlasting—the healing that came when we remembered Shabbat and kept it holy.

■

AFFIRMATION

Each time I observe a Sabbath, I help to heal my body and soul.

■

Remember the Sabbath day, and keep it holy.
EXODUS 20:8

Even the sinners in Hell have rest on the Sabbath.
YIDDISH PROVERB

SELF

*the entire person of an individual; the union of
elements (body, mind, emotions, psyche)*

■

To be what you are, who you are, can't be called a failure.
ANATOLE BROYARD

All acts of healing are ultimately our selves healing our Self.
RAM DASS

There is only one core issue for all psychology. Where is the "me?"
Where does the "me" begin? Where does the "me" stop?
JAMES HILLMAN

THE LATE Edwin H. Friedman, an ordained rabbi, family therapist, and author, wrote fables to create a fresh perspective on human foibles. In "The Bridge," we meet a man who has given much thought to his life. In the process of discerning what he wanted and how he might get it, the man experienced many moods, trials, challenges, setbacks, successes, and failures. Diligently, he searched for the right opportunity, and at last it came. But, he discovered, he must commit himself to claiming it quickly, or it would pass.

Hurrying along, the man came to a very high bridge. As he began crossing, a stranger approached, dressed similarly except for a rope wrapped around his waist. "Pardon me," said the stranger, "would you hold the end of this rope?"

Surprised, the man reached out and took it. Just as he did, the other jumped off the bridge. Instinctively, the man held tight and braced himself. "Why did you do this?" he asked.

"Remember, if you let go, I will be lost," the stranger replied. "I am your responsibility. My life is in your hands, so hang on."

Alas, every attempt the man made to find help and rid himself of his newfound burden failed. Frustrated, he wrapped the rope around *his* waist. If the other lets go, he reasoned, he will be haunted by his actions. If he stays, he will forfeit his journey to salvation. Then, realizing that if he did not remain true to his own goal, he would lose everything, he suddenly knew what he must do.

"Listen carefully," he said while untying the rope around his waist. "I will not accept the position of choice for your life, only for my own. The position of choice for your own life I hereby give back to you. You decide which way this ends. I will become the counterweight. Begin pulling to bring yourself up."

In disbelief, the stranger shrieked, "You cannot mean what you say. You would not be so selfish. I am your responsibility. Do not do this to me."

For a moment, the man stood thoughtfully and noticed that there was no change in the tension of the rope. "I accept your choice," he said. And with that, he freed his hands.

■

AFFIRMATION

I've got to be me.

■

Wherever you go, you can't get rid of yourself.
POLISH PROVERB

Each bay its own wind.
ENGLISH PROVERB

SELF-CONTROL

*restraint exercised over one's impulses,
emotions, or desires*

■

The perfect no-stress environment is the grave.
When we change our perception we gain control.
The stress becomes a challenge, not a threat. When we commit
to action, to actually doing something rather than feeling trapped
by events, the stress in our life becomes manageable.
GREG ANDERSON

When you realize that you have control over any interpretation
you place upon your body, an enormously liberating idea
begins to dawn; the body is on your side.
DEEPAK CHOPRA

A little kingdom I possess,
Where thoughts and feelings swell;
And very hard the task I find
Of governing it well.
LOUISA MAY ALCOTT

BACK IN THE fifties in Brooklyn, New York, the few people in our neighborhood who weren't Jewish were seasonally conspicuous. Christmas lights or Easter decorations were real giveaways. Of course, if you were Black, your differences weren't confined to just holidays. Such was the case with our neighbor Jackie Robinson, the first Black man to play professional baseball.

Although I was too young to be one of the kids on the block who got to root for him regularly from the stands, I was old enough to remember Jackie telling stories about his life. Years later, after his death in 1972, I heard yet another that literally drove home his words to us about the importance of feeling in control of one's self.

As that story goes, when given the opportunity to move from a team in the Negro League into the world of white baseball, Jackie knew it would be an enormous risk that could cost him his career. But crossing that threshold would also be the fulfillment of his vision for his future. Jackie decided to go for it, but not before Dodgers manager Branch Rickey made the rookie first baseman promise that he would never retaliate for insults thrown his way.

As Rickey predicted, each time Jackie played ball, the crowds hurled racial slurs at him. As promised, Jackie fielded the harsh words but never hurled them back. Invariably, his self-control further inflamed the spectators. "Shoeshine boy!" "Black S.O.B." and "Nigger!" they would shout mercilessly. Still, Jackie stayed true to his word—even when some players went beyond verbal abuse.

Enter Dodgers captain PeeWee Reese during a game when taunts flew at Jackie from both the stands and other players. Reese, a Southerner, called time out and walked straight to Jackie. Then, without saying a word, he put his arm around his Black teammate's shoulders and stared—at his opponents and the crowd. Reese's unspoken message flew not only into the dugout, but into the hearts of baseball fans everywhere.

■

AFFIRMATION

More and more I know that when things around me seem out of control,

all I can control is my self

■

I am myself my own commander.
LATIN PROVERB

He is strong who conquers others;
he who conquers himself is mighty.
LAO-TZU

SELF-LOVE

the instinct or desire to promote one's own well-being; regard for or love of one's self

■

If you don't love yourself, you have nothing to hold on to.
BEN VEREEN

Without being and remaining oneself, there is no love.
MARTIN BUBER

Why not fall in love with the body you've been
sleeping with all your life?
STEWART EMERY

NEITHER OF MY parents was a wanted child. While growing up, my father's parents drilled the message into him that he was a loser. My mother fared no better. Her parents made it clear that their lives and marriage would have been much better if they had had only one child—my mother's younger sister. Not surprisingly, when my parents met, each believed the other's love would magically putty all the holes in their hearts. That, of course, never happened, and their marriage ended in divorce.

Afterwards, my mother spent years wallowing in the hatred she felt toward my father. However, she did eventually forgive him for both real and perceived hurts. My father, on the other hand, never forgave my mother. When I asked him why, he blamed her for his disappointments and pain. When I asked my mother why she could forgive a man who had incessantly raged and abused her, she said it was because one day she fell in love with herself. "I hated myself for over sixty years. When I finally decided to stop going there and look for places in me that were lovable, I found hidden treasure—parts of me that overflowed with so much love that I needed to give some of it away. That's when I knew I could forgive your father."

Educator and rabbi Joshua Loth Liebman said it was important for all of us "to become aware of how we become enslaved to false notions of what we are and what we ought to be." He maintained that many times when we think we are loving ourselves we are, in fact, "really strangling or suffocating ourselves with morbid self-concern. We maintain a cruel contempt for our own capabilities and virtues or become unconscious victims of a paralyzing egocentricity."

Liebman says that when we free ourselves from false self-love, which is narcissism, that destructive self-hatred which is masochism, we become friendly with ourselves and others. Then we are on the road to proper self-love, which implies many things. Self-love is rooted in self-respect, he concludes. Furthermore, "no man or woman can have self-respect unless he has learned the art of self-acceptance."

■

AFFIRMATION

More and more I know that I can only love others as I respect,

accept, and love myself.

■

I am myself my own nearest of kin.
LATIN PROVERB

Self loves itself best.
PROVERB

SILENCE

the absence of sound; stillness

■

Who then tells a finer tale than any of us? Silence does.
ISAK DINESEN

Do not the most moving moments of our lives
find us all without words?
MARCEL MARCEAU

What is always speaking silently is the body.
NORMAN O. BROWN

I'M AN INTROVERT who loves the sound of silence. That's why I remember December 1996 was the last time I heard it clearly. By the middle of January 1997, I noticed that whenever I listened for that revered sound, a whistling in my ears supplanted it. So I went to my doctor, who told me I had tinnitus.

Tin•ni•tus—a sound in one ear or both ears, such as buzzing, ringing, or whistling, occurring without an external stimulus and usually caused by a specific condition, such as an ear infection, the use of certain drugs, a blocked auditory tube or canal, or a head injury

"I've never had any of the things that cause this," I told the doctor. "What'll stop it?"

"Nothing," he said. "It's irreversible."

What was the silence that Helen Keller knew? Was it the silence we experience when the sound track suddenly cuts off in a movie? Was it my kind of silence—one that has the gravelly sound of s-s-s-s-s going on and on? Or was it the silence of nothingness—nothing before, nothing after?

Later that year, a group of friends who differed over some issues arrived at our house for a reconciliatory meeting. We put a sign on the door asking them to enter in silence. Not expecting this, some smiled and appeared relieved not to have to talk. Others looked uncomfortable—as if it were a legal gag order. Throughout the evening, we never lifted the ban. For most, dining in silence meant discovering new ways of relating to each other and making their needs known. Conversations that used expressions, eye exchanges, and makeshift sign language said something different than earlier ones filled with angry words and stiff body language. By the time the group got up to leave, they no longer looked ill at ease. Instinctively, as the men and women put on their coats, they began hugging each other good-bye—warm, lasting hugs—body to body and cheek to cheek instead of cursory clutches.

In whatever way our guests experienced silence that night, it created a space that helped to transform anger and deepen their relationships and responses to each other and themselves. That night the sacred sound of silence helped to peacefully usher in a dawn. Silent night. Healing night. All is calm. . . .

■

AFFIRMATION

Silence whispers healing words.

■

Silence is a healing of all ailments.
HEBREW PROVERB

In silence God brings all to pass.
GREEK PROVERB

SMILE

*an upward curving of the corners of the mouth
that indicates pleasure,
amusement, or derision*

■

A smile is a curve that sets everything straight.
PHYLLIS DILLER

Smiles reach the hard-to-reach places.
STEVE WILSON

Let a smile be your umbrella, and you'll get a lot of rain in your face.
GARY RABINOWITZ

DO YOUR SMILES come naturally? Or do you find it easier to frown? Do you have people in your life who can illuminate whole rooms with their effortless, contagious grin? My guess is that if we could be flies on the wall, we'd see them smiling when they're alone—perhaps even through times of deep suffering and pain.

"Even though life is hard, even though it is sometimes difficult to smile, we have to try. Just as when we wish each other, 'Good morning, it must be a real 'Good morning,' " says Thich Nhat Hanh, the Vietnamese Buddhist monk and poet who was nominated for the Nobel Peace Prize. Hanh, who was the chairman of the Vietnamese Buddhist peace delegation during the war, now lives in exile in France and leads retreats worldwide.

Once, when a friend asked him how he could force himself to smile when he was filled with sorrow, Hanh told her that she must be able to smile to her sorrow, because we are more than our sorrow. "A human being is like a television set with millions of channels," he explains in *Being Peace*. "If we turn the Buddha on, we are the Buddha. If we turn sorrow on, we are sorrow. If we turn a smile on, we really are the smile. We cannot let just one channel dominate us. We have the seed of everything in us, and we have to seize the situation in our hand, to recover our own sovereignty."

Our smiles affirm our awareness and determination to live lives filled with peace and joy, Hanh adds. Moreover, when we remember to smile when awakening—even if it takes hanging a reminder such as a branch, a leaf, a painting, or some inspiring words close by—it helps us approach the day with gentleness and understanding. Even the tiniest bud of a smile on our lips has the healing power to relax all the muscles in our face, banish worries and fatigue, nourish awareness, calm us, and return us to the peace we thought we had lost.

AFFIRMATION

I know when I smile it brings happiness to me and those around me.

Every tear has a smile behind it.
IRANIAN PROVERB

Often truth spoken with a smile
will penetrate the mind and reach the heart.
HORACE

SOLITUDE

the state or quality of being alone
or remote from others

■

She would not exchange her solitude for anything. Never again to be
forced to move to the rhythms of others.
TILLIE OLSEN

Inside myself is a place where I live alone and that's where you renew
your springs that never dry up.
PEARL BUCK

Solitude is the furnace of transformation.
HENRI NOUWEN

I GREW UP IN a very noisy household. Few days passed when my parents
didn't find a reason to take their abiding anger out on each other or on
my two sisters and me. So, early on, I discovered that solitude, where and
when I could find it, was a practical place to go to assuage confusion and
pain.

In those early years, the dark, narrow space between our house and our
neighbor's became my hideaway. There, I would slither down between the
cold red bricks and gray mortar to just be. Not until I outgrew that pint-
sized lair did I discover that slithering into solitude like a wounded animal
wasn't my only option. Intentionally entering its domain to experience a
full range of feelings and emotions became another.

Over the years, those with whom I've shared intimate details about my
family of origin have asked how I managed to survive the childhood abuse I
suffered. I believe that the precious gift of solitude that I reaped from my
parents' anger is one, if not *the* answer. Looking back, I realize that early on

I learned that solitude sanctifies. There, in its holy chambers, I discovered there was more to healing than licking my wounds. There I could talk to the heavens and wait, uninterrupted, for answers from a voice deep inside that had something vital to say. There I began to find an "I" that was separate from others. There I felt the difference between being alone and being lonely. There I gathered the strength to know what I stood for and what I could stand up against. Ultimately, solitude taught me what the phrase "the peace that passeth all understanding" might truly mean. And in that peace, I experienced hundreds of deaths and as many resurrections.

At one time I sought the safety of solitude because I feared for my life. Today, I seek the serenity of solitude to renew my life. Once I sought solitude in a hard, cold place to try to gather the shattered pieces of my psyche and soul. Today, like a chick under a mother hen's protective wing, I bask in the warmth I find in solitude, and it reminds me I am whole.

■

AFFIRMATION

The time I give myself for solitude is life-giving.

■

An undisturbed mind is the best salve for affliction.
LATIN PROVERB

Solitude is within us.
FRENCH PROVERB

SOUL

*the immaterial essence, animating principle, or
actuating cause of an individual life*

■

The human body is the best picture of the human soul.
LUDWIG WITTGENSTEIN

A sound and healthy body is dependent on a sound and healthy soul.
MANACHEM MENDEL SCHNEERSON

The soul is not an idea or a belief; it is an experience.
RACHEL NAOMI REMEN

SEVERAL YEARS AGO, psychotherapist Thomas Moore wrote a series of
best-selling books that examined how the soul operates and manifests
itself. For Moore, the soul is not a religious object or some ethereal part of
us that survives our physical death. Instead, the soul is a quality or a dimen-
sion of experiencing life and ourselves that has to do with depth, heart,
value, relatedness, and personal substance.

To care for our soul we must become familiar with its ways, advises
Moore. "Observance is a word from ritual and religion. It means to watch out
for but also to keep and honor, as in the observance of a holiday. The *-serv-* in
observance originally referred to tending sheep. Observing the soul, we keep
an eye on its sheep, on whatever is wandering and grazing—the latest addiction, a striking dream, or a troubling mood."

Caring for the soul also includes not treating it like a self-improvement
project and respecting whatever it presents—even illness. "As a psychotherapist," says Moore, "I won't try to take away the things that bother people in
the name of health." Instead of trying to eradicate the causes of our *dis*ease
like an exterminator, he suggests reflecting on what is problematical and

determining its necessity, even its value. "When you regard the soul with an open mind, you begin to find the messages that lie within the illness, the corrections that can be found in remorse and other uncomfortable feelings, and the necessary changes requested by depression and anxiety."

How, on a day-to-day basis, do we know that we are caring for our soul? According to Moore, it's when compassion takes the place of distrust and fear, when we can let go of the need to be free of complexity and confusion, and when our pleasures feel deeper than usual. "Soul is its own purpose and end."

■

■

Why do you hasten to remove anything which hurts your eye, while if
something affects your soul you postpone the cure until next year?
HORACE

It is more necessary to cure the soul than the body.
GREEK PROVERB

SPIRIT

*an animating or vital principle said to give life
to physical organisms;
the essential nature of a person*

■

It isn't until you come to a spiritual understanding of who you are—not
necessarily a religious feeling, but deep down, the spirit within—that
you can begin to take control.
OPRAH WINFREY

The art of true healing is when you can stimulate
a person's own spirit to shine through.
SANDRA INGERMAN

True spirituality does not exist without love of life.
NATHANIEL BRANDEN

MY ENCOUNTERS WITH people suffering from spiritual *dis*ease go back to
my childhood. Although I would like to believe that experiences span-
ning more than five decades gave me answers to solving the mystery of spiritual healing, the truth is, they haven't. They've only offered me clues.

Worldwide, indigenous people believe that we are spiritual beings on a
human path, not human beings on a spiritual path. Their healers, known as
shamans, say *all* illness is a spiritual problem, because you cannot separate
the human spirit from the mind and the body. We Westerners tend to see
things in reverse. Instead of focusing on the spiritual realm within, we go
on journeys to find it in the outside world. Oftentimes that helps, but not
as expected. As the poet T.S. Eliot reminds us, the boon from such explo-
ration is not what's found abroad. It comes at the journey's end, when we
find ourselves going through an "unknown, remembered gate" to know the
place where we started for the first time.

Looking back, I see many people in my life who never traveled back through that unknown, remembered gate. These were the people whose journeys led them to abuse alcohol, drugs, and food—bottled up, packaged spirits that numbed, drowned, and padded their intractable pain. There were also people whose spiritual quests led them to use religion the same way. Rather than seeing rituals, sacraments, codes of conduct, and religious leaders as keys that could open the gate, they used them as ends in themselves.

More than once, I told a lifelong friend how much I respected her for giving up addictions to alcohol and drugs cold turkey. She hated her life, she confessed, until one night when she dreamt she was at her funeral. "Not one person said anything nice or kind about me. The pain was horrible, and when I tried ignoring it, it got worse. Finally, a voice spoke to me through the pain. All it said was 'God loves you. Love life.'"

When she wakened, my friend swore she would never drink or do drugs again. "I don't know whose voice it was, but it was filled with spirit," she said many times afterwards. "I suspect it's what some call the Holy Spirit, because as soon as it spoke, I knew what it said was true."

■

AFFIRMATION

My spirit is perfect, divine, and healing.

■

A broken spirit is hard to heal.
YIDDISH PROVERB

The spirit illuminates everything.
CHINESE PROVERB

STORY

an account or a recital of an event or a series of events, either true or fictitious

■

We tell tales to heal the soul, for only then can we
begin to heal the body and mind.
EDWARD HOFFMAN

Stories are medicine.
CLARISSA PINKOLA ESTES

Stories give people the feeling that there is meaning, that there is ultimately an order lurking behind the incredible confusion of appear-
ances and phenomena that surrounds them.
WIM WENDERS

WHAT WOULD YOU do if you dreamed your soul was beckoning you to
follow it into maximum security prisons, insane asylums, hospitals,
and dark, litter-strewn alleys? Once upon a time, when Brother Blue had
that dream, he decided that it was divine intervention calling him to be a
storyteller. Today, this slightly built holy fool, who is really Hugh Morgan
Hill, Ph.D., is the official storyteller of Boston, Cambridge, and the United
Nations Habitat Forum. Daily, he dresses in a trademark blue turtleneck
and multicolored jacket and beret adorned with ribbons, balloons, banners,
bells, and his symbol of metamorphosis—butterflies. Then, barefooted, he
heads out to the streets and town squares to hawk healing stories about the
human condition.

Once when I asked Blue why he felt called to help heal broken people's
lives by telling stories, he replied: "The call came to me this way. Once I had
a brother who could not read or write. He had a learning disability. He was

called retarded. I don't like that word. My brother's soul was so bright—who can measure the soul? But I couldn't teach him to read or write. He died in an institution and I made a vow to go all over the world to find those who have problems. I want to tell them stories so they will believe in themselves and know that they're loved."

For twelve years, Blue carried slave chains in his little rainbow bag. He got them from a professor at Harvard whose great-grandfather got them at a slave market during the Civil War. "I carried those chains to remind me there's work to do. You've got to break chains off people, off their minds, off their way of living. A story is a forever thing. We're all messengers. When we tell our stories we turn them into prayers that help us heal one another and bless all life."

■

AFFIRMATION

When I share my healing stories, I bless others in the world around me.

■

A good tale is none the worse for being told twice.
ENGLISH PROVERB

Have nothing to do with profane myths and old wives' tales.
1 TIMOTHY 4:7

STRENGTH

quality or state of being strong

∎

Strength is the capacity to break a chocolate bar into four pieces with
your bare hands—and then eat just one of the pieces.
JUDITH VIORST

I was always looking outside myself for strength and confidence but it
comes from within. It is there all the time.
ANNA FREUD

The first question to be answered by any individual or any social group
facing a hazardous situation is whether the crisis is to be met as a challenge to strength or as an occasion for despair.
HARRY EMERSON FOSDICK

A FABLE BY AESOP tells about a father who despaired because his sons
perpetually quarreled. As the tale goes:

When the father failed to heal their disputes by his exhortations, he told
them to fetch a bundle of sticks. He then placed it into the hands of each of
them in succession and ordered them to break it in pieces. They tried with
all their strength, but were not able to do it. Next, he opened the bundle and
put a single stick into each son's hands. They broke easily. He then said: "My
sons, if you are of one mind, and unite to assist each other, you will be as this
bundle, uninjured by all the attempts of your enemies; but if you are divid-
ed among yourselves, you will be broken as easily as these sticks."

According to my friend, Bud a gifted musician and recovering alcoholic,
our cultural imperative to "be strong" can be misleading. "Whenever I felt
really strong I wanted a drink," he said. "But it took being weak to know that

my life needed to change." Bud also told me that the place where he felt the weakest was when he finally hit bottom. "But how did you know when you hit it?" I asked. "You hit bottom when you stop digging," he replied.

Of course, not all of us dig ourselves into holes and despair. Sometimes we fall in because of accidents, illnesses, or uncontrollable circumstances. But no matter how we got in, we must begin to heal the wounds to our bodies, psyches, or souls to get out. Both Bud and Aesop offer similar advice. If you can't get yourself out of the hole, hold the hands of others who have already pooled their strength and can show you the way. On the way out, take just one step at a time. They're cumulative. And also believe that your real strength lies in knowing when to hang on and when to let go; when to trust yourself and when to trust others—both human and Divine.

■

AFFIRMATION

My weaknesses help teach me what I need to become strong.

■

My strength is made perfect in weakness.
CORINTHIANS

The burden is equal to the horse's strength.
TALMUD

SURRENDER

the act of yielding one's person; to give back

■

The healing process is made up of unconditional love,
forgiveness, and letting go of fear.
GERALD JAMPOLSKY

If you surrendered to the air you could ride it.
TONI MORRISON

At fifteen life had taught me, undeniably, that surrender, in its place,
was as honorable as resistance, especially if one had no choice.
MAYA ANGELOU

TO SOME, THE word *surrender* conjures up negative images of capitulation. For others, such as someone letting go of an unhealthy behavior, the word feels more positive. In either case, when we surrender to something or someone, it implies that we admit to being or feeling powerless to change anything but ourselves.

I believe all of us know something about that feeling. As children there were always times we had to surrender pieces of our person. Sometimes we did so willingly to parents and others in whom we placed our trust. Other times, we surrendered to overpowering forces—perhaps schoolyard bullies, institutions, or illnesses. Indeed, as I look back on what I have surrendered during my lifetime, it strikes me that when we admit to ourselves that we are powerless under certain circumstances, our confession is not just a function of the ego but of the heart.

The car accident that permanently disabled Ted's son Chris happened four years before we met. Besides massive head injuries, Chris, now thirty, suffered broken bones in every limb in his body and lay unconscious in a coma for a month. Doctors did not expect the red-haired, freckle-faced thirteen-year-old to live. To keep watch over their son, brother, and grandson, Chris's family camped at the hospital. Invariably, Ted would always arrive impeccably dressed in a suit and tie. With each visit, he brought renewed hope that he would find Chris awake and on the road to recovery. With each departure, he knew that all he could do was to continue to cling to his hope and pray he could somehow will God to answer his prayers.

One evening, as he arrived for his "watch," Ted passed a mirror. Looking at the man in a dark suit reflected back, Ted peered into a stranger's eyes. Shocked, he shed his jacket and tie, unbuttoned his stiff starched shirt, and rolled up his sleeves. "I felt raw when I entered Chris's room. I sat down beside him and began crying. Then I began praying from a place in my heart that I hadn't felt in a long, long time. 'Thy will be done. . . . Thy will be done.'"

■

AFFIRMATION

When I surrender my armor, I open my heart.

■

Better indeed is knowledge than mechanical practice. Better than knowledge is meditation. But better still is surrender of attachment to results, because there follows immediate peace.
BHAGAVAD GITA

Love conquers all, let us surrender to love.
VIRGIL

TEARS

*secretions that overflow the eyelids and dampen
the face; an act of weeping or grieving*

■

There is a sacredness in tears.
They speak more eloquently than ten thousand tongues.
WASHINGTON IRVING

The sorrow which has no vent in tears may make other organs weep.
HENRY HAUDSLEY

The soul would have no rainbow had the eyes no tears.
JOHN VANCE CHENEY

I DIDN'T CRY WHEN my father died. When I was a child, this man, who would never allow me to get close to him, always admonished me not to cry. So I didn't. Not so when my mother died. Although there had been a time when I felt very distant from her, that hour had long passed. By both our choices, we had become very close, and my tears of remembrance still unabashedly flow. Sometimes my tears help to dilute the sorrow and lingering pain I feel. Sometimes they cleanse places in my heart and soul that harbor messy memories best forgotten, while other times they rise in response to warm, loving ones. Always they bring the reassurance and relief that I had no unfinished business with her. Always they remind me that when someone dies, that relationship is left forever wherever it was left.

The night before Mom died in the hospital, she was comatose. The ventilator tube that passed through her lips and into her throat mechanically inhaled and exhaled for her. After a long bedside vigil, my sisters and I got up to get a bite to eat. "I'll be back real soon, Mom," I said while bending over to kiss her forehead. Suddenly, with her eyes still shut, it looked as though she was trying to acknowledge me. "Mom, can you hear me?" Again it seemed she could.

For the next fifteen minutes, Bobbi, Deborah, and I took turns standing beside the woman who brought us into this world and spoke words of love and gratitude as she departed. With each change of voice, Mom gave some small indication that she knew who was there, until suddenly she drifted back into the depths of an abiding sleep. Looking at my sisters, I said, "She may never be able to be with us again." Looking back at Mom, we discovered one pearllike tear glistening in the corner of her eye.

Listen solicitously
to sudden surprise tears
that shove to the surface
all unexpectedly—
set off by dear knows what—
a sound, a gesture,
a song, a sigh,
and there you are, all shaken
to the very depths.
SADIE M. GREGORY

■

AFFIRMATION

My tears help me cross the valley of the shadow of death.

■

There is a palace that opens only to tears.
ZOHAR

A tear in place is better than a smile out of place.
IRANIAN PROVERB

THOUGHTS

a product of thinking

■

Great thoughts reduced to practice become great acts.
WILLIAM HAZLITT

There is a criterion by which you can judge whether the thoughts you
are thinking are right for you. The criterion is:
Have they brought you inner peace? If not, there is
something wrong with them—so keep seeking!
PEACE PILGRIM

Nothing is good or bad but thinking makes it so.
WILLIAM SHAKESPEARE

DURING THOSE TIMES when we feel ill at ease with the world or ourselves, our thoughts tend to wander. In *The Soul's Almanac,* interfaith minister Aaron Zerah retells a traditional Hindu tale that describes the power those itinerant thoughts can have over us. As the story opens, we meet a man who wandered throughout the world in search of his deepest desire. However, despite looking everywhere, he could never find the happiness and fulfillment he sought. Finally, one day, tired from his search, he sat down underneath a great tree. What he did not know was that this was the Great Wish-Fulfilling Tree. Whatever one wishes for when seated underneath it immediately becomes true.

While resting in his weariness, the man thought to himself, "What a beautiful spot this is. I wish I had a home here," and instantly before his eyes a home appeared. Delighted, he thought further, "Ah, if only I had a partner to be here with me, then my happiness would be complete," and in a moment a beautiful woman calling him "husband" was manifested. Before going to her, he thought about his hunger, wishing to satisfy it, and immediately a banquet table appeared, covered with every kind of food and drink. Then, while feasting hungrily, the man thought, "I wish I had a servant to serve me the rest of this food." Instantly, one appeared.

Upon finishing the meal, the man sat against the wonderful tree and began to reflect, "How amazing. Everything I wished has come true. There is some mysterious force about this tree. I wonder if there is a demon who lives in it?" As soon as he finished asking himself the question, a great demon appeared. "Oh, my," he thought, "this demon will probably eat me up," and so it did.

■

AFFIRMATION

My positive thoughts help manifest health, happiness, and healing.

■

If you want to see what your thoughts were like yesterday, look at your
body today. If you want to see what your body will be like tomorrow,
look at your thoughts today.
INDIAN PROVERB

We are what we think. All that we are arises with out thoughts.
With our thoughts we make the world.
THE BUDDHA

TIME

the measured or measurable period
during which an action, process,
or condition exists or continues

■

Time is a dressmaker specializing in alterations.
FAITH BALDWIN

Time does not heal. But healing does take time.
DEBORAH MORRIS CORYELL

Don't serve time, let time serve you.
ANNA M. KROSS (TO PRISON INMATES)

ARE YOU LIKE millions of other people who suffer from time pressure and time sickness? Do you find yourself stressed from trying to keep time from marching on, slipping by, flying away, ticking away, or running out? Do you worry about the ways in which you spend time, mark time, waste time, and lose time? Do you try to steal, borrow, or buy time as if it were a commodity? When was the last time your remember feeling that time stood still, or that it was manageable, or that it wasn't disappearing?

We all know the saying "Time heals all wounds," but is that a realistic expectation for those of us who suffer from an addiction to juggling time or time stress? How can we change our perception that we're in a time famine? How can we shift gears so that we sit in the driver's seat and time no longer drives us?

Author John Steinbeck wondered, too. "Where does the discontent start?" he asked. "You are warm enough, but you shiver. You are fed, yet hunger gnaws at you. You have been loved, but your yearning wanders in new fields. And to prod all these there's time, the Bastard Time."

Stephen Rechtschaffen, M.D., cofounder of the Omega Institute for Holistic Health, which is the nation's largest holistic learning center, says the antidote for the discontent that accompanies time sickness is timeshifting. He explains that timeshifting, instead of time management, is a technique for synchronizing the rhythms in our inner and outer worlds that helps us to feel more balanced. We learn to choose active and positive responses to time pressure and anxiety instead of merely reacting to it, either passively or negatively. We become mindful of our thoughts and emotional states and speed up or slow down the pace of our lives in response to what's happening to us.

Answering the telephone illustrates this. When this "time thief" rings, are you someone who lunges for the receiver? Buddhist monk and Zen master Thich Nhat Hanh suggests a timeshifting alternative. Instead of reacting, respond so you can make a shift from what you were doing. First, pause and allow the phone to ring three times. While it does, take three deep breaths to become focused. Then pick it up. Instead of feeling stressed and interrupted, you will probably feel more relaxed and present to the person on the other end. You may even discover you're smiling.

■

AFFIRMATION

I make time my ally when I live in the present moment.

■

Time will bring healing.
GREEK PROVERB

Time is the best doctor.
YIDDISH PROVERB

TOUCH

*to perceive by the sense of feeling; to lay hands
on; to affect; to arouse an emotion in*

■

There is a mysterious healing power in touch that is beyond words and
beyond our ideas about it.
AILEEN CROW

Often the hands will solve a mystery that the intellect has struggled
with in vain.
CARL JUNG

You need four hugs a day for survival, eight for maintenance and
twelve for growth.
VIRGINIA SATIR

NOTHING WILL EVER erase the memory of the moment I touched my
breast and felt a lump. As I stood in the shower doing my version of
the monthly self-examination recommended by the American Cancer
Society, the tips of my fingers moved across familiar terrain. "It almost
seems silly to be doing this," I thought. "You just had a clean mammogram
seven weeks ago." But habits being what habits are, when the right side felt
free and clear, I moved over to the left. Once again, my fingers began a Tour
de Breast in concentric circles. "Nothing doing," I sighed after taking a necessary sharp turn into my armpit. "Almost done. One more round—a little
harder this time to doublecheck."

Just as I was about to cross the finish line, I felt *it* lying next to my breast
bone. A wave of fear washed over the furthest reaches of my inner space.
"Couldn't be," I said as my stomach flipped a hundred and eighty degrees.
Several touches later, I still expected something to change. Nothing did.

Immediately, I notified my intruder that it had twenty-four hours to evacuate the premises. A day later, as I stood in the shower damning it for not following instructions, I accepted the fact that an alien invader had claimed squatter's rights in my body. Hours later, in my gynecologist's office, he confirmed *it* wasn't a figment of my imagination. And as much as we both wanted the tiny, malleable lump to be a harmless cyst, tests proved otherwise.

Two days after my lumpectomy, I showered for the first time. With trepidation, I eased the left side of my body into the stream of water. Instead of hurting, the warm, cleansing drops felt healing as they touched my skin. Later, I headed over to Ted's church for Sunday services. As I reentered the unique community that has hands-on ministries to help those with AIDS, the homeless, gay men and women, and other marginalized people, I was infused with its healing spirit. Friends and strangers greeted me with care-filled embraces that carefully avoided my left side. Their encouraging words of support filled my heart, and the healing prayers they offered for my health and well-being touched the deepest recesses of my soul.

■

AFFIRMATION

What touches me can help to heal me.

■

He will deliver you from six troubles;
in seven no harm shall touch you.
JOB 5:19

And all in the crowd were trying to touch him, for power came out from
him and healed all of them.
LUKE 6:19

TRUST

firm reliance on the integrity, ability,
or character of a person or thing;
reliance on something in the future

■

Trust yourself, then you will know how to live.
JOHANN WOLFGANG VON GOETHE

Trust what moves you most deeply.
SAM KEEN

Trust life, and it will teach you, in joy and sorrow,
all you need to know.
JAMES BALDWIN

LIKE MANY LONG-MARRIED couples in their eighties, Hugh and Naftel found themselves relying more and more on each other as their minds and bodies began to fail them. Naftel, who always prided herself on having the sharp memory every good teacher needed, found words slipping away and missing. As the problem grew worse, she trusted Hugh to speak up and fill in the gaps. In turn, as Hugh's eyesight began failing him, he placed more and more trust in Naftel to safely guide him through the day and into bed at night. Their mutual trust became especially important when they at last had to leave their familiar home and live in an apartment in a senior housing complex.

One day, Hugh learned that a big band would be playing that evening at the complex. When he asked his bride of so many years if she would like to dine and dance, she eagerly said yes. That night, as they moved to the music of their youth, Hugh and Naftel's infirmities seemed to fade. Hugh's feet went on autopilot as he guided her across the dance floor, and Naftel trusted him to get her where they were going. And as the familiar tunes jogged her memory of other dances they had shared, she recalled the most memorable ones without Hugh having to fill in a word.

When the music ended, both Hugh and Naftel again turned to each other for support. On the way back to their apartment, she took the lead and he helped her find words to express how much she enjoyed the evening. Once inside, they sat down on the couch. Hugh thanked Naftel for all their years together. Naftel did the same, and then, as she put her head on her trusted partner's shoulder, she died.

From the cradle to the grave, life teaches us who and what outside ourselves we can trust and why. Perhaps the lesson is simpler than we often make it out to be. Trust those who have safely guided us from one place to another and those who unconditionally help us to be all we can be to others and ourselves in sickness and in health.

■

AFFIRMATION

Today I will be grateful for those worthy of my trust.

■

In trust is truth.
PROVERB

Some patients, though conscious that their condition is perilous, recover their health simply through their contentment with the goodness of the physician.
HIPPOCRATES

TRUTH

conformity to fact or actuality; reality

■

It always comes back to the same necessity: go deep enough and there
is a bedrock of truth, however hard.
MAY SARTON

There are times when we must sink to the bottom of our misery to
understand truth, just as we must descend to the bottom of a well
to see the stars in broad daylight.
VÁCLAV HAVEL

The best mind-altering drug is truth,
LILY TOMLIN

A STORY ABOUT JESUS speaks of a woman who hemorrhaged for twelve
years and spent all her money on physicians. But, alas, they were not able
to stop her flow of blood, which grew progressively worse. When she heard
Jesus was in town, the desperate woman thought, "If I can just touch his
clothes, I will be made well." So she made her way through the crowd and
touched his garment from behind. Immediately, her hemorrhage stopped.

Jesus, aware that something had happened, turned around. "Who
touched my clothes?" he asked. His disciples replied, "You see the crowd
pressing in on you; how can you ask, 'Who touched me?' " But the woman,
knowing what had happened, came in fear and trembling and told him the
whole truth. After listening, Jesus then told her to go in peace—that her
faith had made her well and healed her of her disease.

Every time I read that story I'm struck by the words *whole truth*. What, I
wonder, does it mean to tell the whole truth? What's the difference between
not lying and telling the whole truth? Is it when I spill every last fact? Is it a
feeling of congruency in my inner and outer worlds? Does it mean including

all—not only those parts of me which are attractive, beautiful, appealing, and good, but those that are repulsive, ugly, unappealing, and evil, too? What happens inside me when I speak one truth but intuitively feel that something else is *the* truth? Does it matter, as long as no one gets hurt? What is it about not telling the whole truth to others and myself that keeps me from being healed? What is it about the whole truth that allows us to feel well and be healed?

"The condition of truth is to let suffering speak," says Harvard professor and African-American intellectual Cornel West. Whether or not the story about the encounter between the woman with the flow of blood and Jesus is literally true doesn't matter to me. What does matter is what it tells us about the healing we can all experience when our suffering speaks its whole truth.

■

AFFIRMATION

More and more I know the healing power of the whole truth.

■

Be a lamp to yourself. Be your own confidence. Hold to the truth within
yourself, as to the only truth.
THE BUDDHA

You will know the truth, and the truth will make you free.
JOHN THE EVANGELIST

VOICE

a medium or an agency of expression;
the right or opportunity to express a choice
or an opinion

■

The body is truly the garment of the soul, which has a living voice; for
that reason it is fitting that the body, simultaneously with the soul,
repeatedly sing praises to God through the voice.
HILDEGARDE VON BINGEN

All cures are partly "talking cures," in Freud's phrase. Every patient
needs mouth-to-mouth resuscitation, for talk is the kiss of life.
ANATOLE BROYARD

Through working with the voice we can learn to enter the state the
Tibetans know as *rigpa*—the awareness which combines emptiness with
clarity. This leads ultimately to illumination.
JILL PURCE

HAVE YOU EVER felt that somewhere in your past someone or something stole your natural voice—the one that would spontaneously
express your thoughts, joy, sorrow, and song? Perhaps it was a parent or a
teacher who told you to be quiet when you were trying to explain or
describe something. Maybe it was when someone said "Don't sing." Possibly
it happened because someone you loved or respected angrily said "Be
silent," "Shut up!" "You're stupid," or other caustic words that silenced you.

In the early nineties, I attended a workshop designed to help me reclaim
the voice my parents stole from me during my childhood. This form of
"soulwork" interested me because I knew that indigenous people had always
used sound as an instrument of healing, and for years I had yearned for my

natural sound, not just my writing, to speak for me. Similar experiences drew others who, like me, were seeking ways to tune in to the sacred sounds in our bodies and help them break through sealed trapdoors in our throats.

By the week's end, many of us felt reunited with a long lost and beloved part of ourselves. This seemed especially true for a withdrawn young woman with a disfiguring harelip. Throughout the week, she sat silently whenever forty-five of us gathered to inhale deeply and then release sonorous sounds as we exhaled. That is, until the last session, when suddenly she stepped into the center of the circle. Anxiously, I watched as she began to rhythmically breathe. With each cycle, her thin body expanded and her mouth opened wider and wider. Then, magically, celestial sounds began floating everywhere. Twenty minutes later, as the sound drifted away, a beautiful, radiant, and confident woman stood before us. I sat stunned by her courage and felt honored to witness the healing power of her voice. Later, she confessed that she had never sung before. "I tried once in the shower a very long time ago," she said. "But I got so scared I never tried again."

■

AFFIRMATION

My natural voice is an instrument of healing.

■

Out of the abundance of the heart the mouth speaks.
MATTHEW 12:34

He who sings frightens away all his ills.
AMERICAN PROVERB

WELLNESS

the quality or state of good
physical and mental health

■

Each of us has a remarkable capacity for self-healing.
However, we have to be the ones to tap it.
STEPHAN RECHTSCHAFFEN

The concept of total wellness recognizes that our every
thought, word, and behavior affects our greater health
and well-being. And we, in turn, are affected not only emotionally but
also physically and spiritually.
GREG ANDERSON

Our bodies are our gardens, to which our wills are our gardeners.
WILLIAM SHAKESPEARE

I N THE LATE nineties, I wrote a book about wellness for a well-known physician. During the planning stage, both of us knew that painting a picture of
the word wellness was going to be tough. Although it's a noun, wellness doesn't
summon up an image like "car" or "toothbrush" or "tree." Instead, it's an intangible quality or condition that lacks a specific form. Yet, we always want to have
it function in our lives. So what does a picture of wellness look like?

Once published, the book offered an excellent representation. However,
for me, something about my picture still felt incomplete. It wasn't until two
years later when breast cancer changed some of my perspectives on wellness
that I finally understood what was missing. First, my experience taught me,
wellness is not the opposite of illness. Moreover, it appears to be a dynamic
form of grace that is a byproduct of being proactive about one's health. Sadly,
some schools of New Age gobbledygook have led many people to believe they

should blame themselves for their diseases – that we cause our cancer or heart attack. Nonsense! We are responsible *to* our health – not for our illnesses. In other words, we are enjoined to be good stewards of our well-being by taking a preventive and holistic approach to our health and being honest enough not to make excuses, justify or rationalize our passivity when we don't.

Shortly after my surgery and radiation treatments, I began to feel much better physically. Yet, intuitively I knew that I was not well. Emotionally, I felt depressed, and the expression, "Things are better than they used to be," became relative. That's when I discovered that if I only concentrated on some "thing" in my life getting better, eventually some other "thing" would get worse. Indeed, some weeks, I felt as though I was a ratchet. First, I'd move two or three steps forward—away from what physically, emotionally, or spiritually felt out of balance—and then, as I eased up on my intention and took my "better" health for granted, I would slide backwards.

Ultimately, my experiences helped me to discern the difference between getting better and getting well. Wellness, I now know, is not about living in the *status quo*. Instead, wellness is about my willingness to balance and then, as things change, rebalance my healthcare equation. It's also about embarking, consciously, on a life-long self-healing journey towards wholeness, and acknowledging that to be a picture of wellness, I must take responsibility for painting it myself.

■

To be a picture of wellness, I must paint it myself.

■

It is better to prevent than to cure.
PERUVIAN

To wish to be well is part of becoming well.
SENECA

WHOLE

containing all components; complete

■

I'm not OK, you're not OK—and that's OK.
WILLIAM SLOANE COFFIN

May the circle be unbroken.
SONG

Of all the needs a lonely child has, the one that must be satisfied, if
there is going to be hope and a hope of wholeness, is the unshaken
need for an unshakable God.
MAYA ANGELOU

MEN, WOMEN, AND children from all walks of life attend services at
Ted's church, and some travel as much as 150 miles round-trip. What
attracts these spiritual seekers to this nationally acclaimed community is its
inclusivity, diversity, and invitation to gather on common ground. St.
Mark's welcomes all to "come as they are." Here, permission need not be
asked to experience or believe in one's God, the Divine, the One, the Holy,
the Creator, Mother, or Father in whatever way one feels is right.

Often, those entering the sanctuary feel less than whole. Several live
with cancer, HIV/AIDS, lupus, heart disease, and other life-threatening diseases. Others endure chronic depression, addictions, arthritis, and mental
illness. The homeless, who come carrying their whole world in plastic bags,
suffer from societal ills, as do many of the people of color and those with
nonconventional sexual orientations.

Although one parishioner named David is in his late forties, he looks like
a little boy. "His pituitary gland doesn't function properly and he just never
grew," explains his mother. As a result, David suffers from multiple disabilities. He wears very thick glasses. He waddles when he walks, and his very

low IQ profoundly limits his speech and comprehension. Yet, she adds, he always asks to go to church, because there he finds a connection to life that he can't find elsewhere. Of equal importance, says Ted, is the way that David has found a niche at St. Mark's and fits in. "At the end of the service, you can hear the whole community silently applauding as his voice rises loudly above everyone else's saying, 'Thanks be to God.' "

In one of Shel Silverstein's children's books, a circle lacking a pie-shaped wedge goes in search of its missing piece. It wants more than anything else to be whole. I believe that's why the people of St. Mark's keep coming together. As they gather in a safe circle on common ground, each discovers that there are no missing pieces.

■

AFFIRMATION

I am who I am. I am whole.

■

Now a whole is that which has a beginning, a middle, and an end.
ARISTOTLE

It is good to sleep in a whole skin.
RUSSIAN PROVERB

WILL

*the mental faculty by which one
deliberately chooses or decides upon
a course of action; volition*

■

**[In sickness] your heaviest artillery will be your will to live.
Keep that big gun going.**
NORMAN COUSINS

**Living had got to be such a habit with him that he
couldn't conceive of any other condition.**
FLANNERY O'CONNOR

**Strength does not come from physical capacity.
It comes from an indomitable will.**
MAHATMA GANDHI

I N "The Secret Sits," poet Robert Frost wrote:

> We dance round in a ring and suppose.
> But the Secret sits in the middle and knows.

That, to me, is what the human will to live feels like—a great big secret
that I can dance around but never reach out and touch; an intangible élan
vital that's indescribable, yet recognizable.

My father spent most of his life working in his hot, grimy boiler shop.
Daily this robust and handsome man left for work in darkness. Late at night
he would return covered with soot. All he cared about was making lots of
money, which he did. He rarely smiled. He never laughed. He seldom saw

his family. He had no time for travel. And if he ever cried for things to be different, we never knew it.

One day my father lost his will to live. He never said that or used those words, but he made it known to all when he got into bed and never got out again. No one could convince him otherwise, and so a caregiver was hired to attend to his personal needs. Lying or sitting on his king-sized throne, he would eat, get bathed, relieve himself, meet with visitors, sleep, phone people, play solitaire, read, and watch television. The first year, one by one, his daughters, other relatives, his acquaintances, his rabbi, and his doctor circled his bed and tried to figure out what prompted his mysterious decision. Was it fear? Was it depression? Was it a cry for attention? Each question, it seemed, contained some truth, but the real reason why his will to live departed remained a secret—even, he said, to him. During the second and third years of his self-imposed exile, everyone gave up trying to figure it out. When he finally did become ill and was diagnosed with colon cancer, he refused treatment.

"What would you do differently?" I asked during my last visit.

"Be willing to love life," he answered as tears welled in his eyes.

■

AFFIRMATION

My love of life affirms my will to live.

■

Will is power.
FRENCH PROVERB

Where there's a will there's a way.
ENGLISH PROVERB

WISDOM

*understanding of what is true, right, or lasting; a
wise outlook, plan, or course of action*

■

One cannot have wisdom without living life.
DOROTHY MCCALL

Wisdom comes through the meeting of the heart and the intellect.
OSHO

My belief is in the blood and flesh as being wiser than the intellect.
D.H. LAWRENCE

MANY YEARS BEFORE she wrote *Discovering the Body's Wisdom,* Mirka
Knaster paid the cost of not listening to what her own body had to
say. Despite the fact that her body kept trying to tell the acclaimed health
writer what *it* needed and wanted, Mirka's mind overrode its messages.
That pattern changed, however, when she literally hit bottom after falling
down a flight of stairs in Asia. Lying in the healing waters of a mountain hot
spring in the Philippines, exhausted from being on the road for a year to do
on-site research on cross-cultural healing arts, she knew, instinctively, that
her body was saying "Go home." Although Mirka listened, it was not long
before her intense drive to know more, be more, and write more kicked in
again.

"People thought I was taking great care of myself—a strict vegetarian who
exercised, meditated, and did all the 'right' things," she says. "But I was living
so much in my head that I had become oblivious to the fact that my body was
screaming 'Stop!' " Finally, while literally lying flat on her back with an inex-
plicable upper respiratory infection, Mirka began listening to her heart, which
all along had been trying to tell her what her head couldn't: that she needed to

shift her attitudes about being a lone ranger and risk sharing her life with another.

Reflecting, Mirka now believes that, although all of us have the wisdom we need to self-heal, it takes more than just collecting "knowledge" to acquire it. Wisdom is a by-product of experiential learning, she says. For example, it's one thing to read about the death of a loved one and feelings associated with that event. It is quite another for our hearts, minds, and souls to feel the pain and grief that accompany that loss. When they do, we become more in touch with ourselves and all humanity. "Our bodies contain a well of ancient wisdom. Our task is to make time to draw from it and drink its healing waters."

> It is good knowing that glasses
> are to drink from;
> the bad thing is not to know
> what thirst is for.
> ANTONIO MACHADO *(trans. Robert Bly)*

■

AFFIRMATION

I help heal my body when I honor its wisdom.

■

Wisdom is to the soul what health is to the body.
FRENCH PROVERB

There is often wisdom under a shabby cloak.
LATIN PROVERB

WORDS

the sounds, combination of sounds,
or representation in writing that symbolizes and
communicates a meaning

■

Words are, of course, the most powerful drug used by mankind.
RUDYARD KIPLING

When the desire to ease someone else's pain is sufficiently deep, one
can almost always find words that will make a difference.
JOSEPH TELUSHKIN

There is one singular ingredient of the art of healing
that should not be allowed to vanish . . .
the transmission of a few encouraging words.
SHERWIN B. NULAND

GROWING UP, MOST of us have experienced the pain of words that maim
and the power of words that heal. Sometimes the intent isn't to do one
or the other. However, once heard or read, words often take on a life of
their own. In *The Lost Art of Healing,* cardiologist Bernard Lown, M.D., tells
stories about words that both harmed and healed his patients.

According to Lown, Mrs. S., forty, had been a heart patient ever since a
childhood bout with acute rheumatic fever damaged her tricuspid valve.
During one hospital stay, her revered physician of thirty years entered her
room to check her condition. Instead of giving Mrs. S. the considerate
attention he usually did, this time he just hurriedly turned to his students
and announced that this was a case of TS.

Afterwards, Lown noticed Mrs. S. was morose. When asked why, she
told him that she thought TS meant "terminal situation." No, he replied. It

means "tricuspid stenosis." Sadly, his words offered no reassurance. Within hours, Mrs. S.'s condition worsened, and early that evening, as Lown stood "transfixed, helpless, and aghast," she died of congestive heart failure. "Such congestion is invariably the result of a failing left ventricle, but her left ventricle was not diseased," he noted.

Years later, Lown was caring for a sixty-year-old man with a grim prognosis. Two weeks earlier, a heart attack had destroyed half of the man's heart muscle, and Lown expected him to die. Instead, the man suddenly recovered.

Six months later, during a follow-up visit, Lown proclaimed the man's recovery a miracle. The man felt otherwise—that it was mind over matter—and explained that one morning when Lown put his stethoscope on the man's chest, he made reference to a "wholesome gallop." "I figured that if my heart was still capable of a healthy gallop, I couldn't be dying, and I got well."

Reflecting on what he considered to be his most remarkable experience in prolonging life, Lown noted, "The patient was unaware that a gallop was a bad sign. A wholesome gallop is an oxymoron. Few remedies are more powerful than a carefully chosen word. Even when the outlook is doubtful, affirmative words promote well-being if not always recovery."

■

AFFIRMATION

When I choose my words carefully, they can help heal others and myself.

■

Words are the voice of the heart.
CHINESE PROVERB

Pleasant words are . . . health to the bones.
PROVERBS 16:24

Afterword

■

Yes!

■

I don't know Who—or what—put the question, I don't know when it was put. I don't even remember answering. But at some moment I did answer Yes to Someone—or Something—and from that hour I was certain that existence is meaningful and that, therefore, my life, in self-surrender, had a goal.

DAG HAMMARSKJÖLD

Yes!

■

Acknowledgments

■

AFTER WRITING AN entire book on the power of words to help heal and transform our lives, I'm at a loss to find all the ones I need to thank everyone who believed in the healing and helping potential of this project and helped make it possible.

From the time the muse awakened me to the idea for *Healing Words*, my agent Ling Lucas encouraged me to stop talking about it and get a proposal down on paper. When I finally did, she wasted no time finding a publisher who she believed would see the healing qualities this project could offer others.

Enter Matthew Lore, my wonderful editor at Marlowe & Company, who offered wise words of his own as the development of the book got underway. Throughout the writing and editing process, Matthew's professionalism, skill, and instincts have guided and inspired me.

Others, to whom I offer my sincere appreciation, include:

Edgar Staren, M.D., Ph.D., Lou Weinstein, M.D., Iman Mohamed, M.D., and John Feldmeir, D.O. After being diagnosed with breast cancer, all four of these skilled physicians not only listened well to the words that tumbled out of my mouth as I sought to understand and grasp the ramifications of the disease, but also proved that there are still doctors who choose to practice healing as an art.

My dear friend Belleruth Naparstek, who not only ordered me to "Get going" when I told her about my ideas for the book, but graciously agreed to write an inspiring foreword as well.

Those who shared their healing stories with me, especially my friends

Cynthia Gale, Deforia Lane, Faye Sholiton, Mary Verdi-Fletcher, Grace Marcotte, Mike Marcotte, Dan Pollock, Bud Roach, Libby Green, Steve Miceli, Laurie Hoeffel, Mirka Knaster, Sandy Ingerman, the women in my healing circle, and all the people at St. Mark's Episcopal Church who have been and continue to be a true source of inspiration and healing for me.

My mentors: The late Arnold Tversky, Verne Edwards, and the Rev. Bill Dols.

Millie, Jane, and Kirk, for being cheerleaders from afar.

Jamie, Evan, Trace, Chris, Terry, and Andie—my beautiful "kids," daughter-in-law, and granddaughter, who bless me over and over again by putting all 101 healing words—especially *forgiveness* and *love*—into action.

And then there's Ted. It would take another book of words for me to express how much I appreciate his love, encouragement, trustworthiness, kindness, companionship, and willingness to give up down time at Berkana so that I could meet my deadlines. Recently, when I looked up the definition of the term *soul mate* in my dictionaries, I found this extraordinary man's picture alongside it.

L'Chayim!

Caren Goldman
Holland, Ohio
January 31, 2001

Bibliography

∎

THE FOLLOWING BOOKS, audiotapes, and worldwide websites were either mentioned by title or used as primary resources for *Healing Words*.

Albert, Susan Wittig. *Writing from Life*. New York: Tarcher/Putnam, 1996.

Allen, Jessica, ed. *Quotable Men of the 20th Century*. New York: Bill Adler Books, 1999.

The American Heritage Dictionary of the English Language 3rd ed. (electronic ed). New York: Houghton Mifflin, 1994.

Anderson, Greg. *Healing Wisdom*. New York: Dutton, 1994.

Andrews, Robert. *Cassell Dictionary of Contemporary Quotations*. London: Cassell Wellington House, 1999.

Augarde, Tony. *The Oxford Dictionary of Modern Quotations*. Oxford: Oxford University Press, 1991

Bartlett, John. *Familiar Quotations*, 14th ed. Boston: Little Brown & Company, 1968.

Beyondananda, Swami. *Duck Soup for the Soul*. Naperville, Ill.: Hysteria Publications, 1999.

Bolen, Jean Shinoda. *Close to the Bone*. New York: Scribner, 1996.

Brallier, Jess M. *Medical Wit and Wisdom*. Philadelphia: Running Press, 1993.

Broyard, Anatole. *Intoxicated by My Illness*. New York: Fawcett, 1993.

Brussat, Frederic, and Mary Ann Brussat, eds. *100 Ways to Keep Your Soul Alive*. San Francisco: HarperSanFrancisco, 1994.

———— *100 More Ways to Keep Your Soul Alive*. San Francisco: HarperSanFrancisco, 1997.

———— *Spiritual Literacy: Reading the Sacred in Everyday Life*. New York: Scribner, 1996.

Brussell, Eugene E. *Webster's New World Dictionary of Quotable Definitions*. Paramus, N.J., Prentice Hall, 1988.

Camp, Wesley D. *Word Lover's Book of Unfamiliar Quotations*. Paramus, N.J., Prentice Hall, 1990.

Campbell, Don G. *The Roar of Silence: Healing Powers of Breath, Tone and Music*. Wheaton, Ill., Quest Books, 1989.

Carlson, Richard, ed. *Healers on Healing*. Los Angeles: J.P. Tarcher, 1989.

Chester, Laura. *Lupus Novice*. Barrytown, N.Y.: Station Hill Press, 1987.

Chopra, Deepak. *Journey into Healing*. New York: Harmony Books, 1994.

Cook, John. *The Book of Positive Quotations*. Minneapolis, Minn., Rubicon Press, 1993.

Coryell, Deborah Morris. *Good Grief: Healing through the Shadow of Loss*. Santa Fe, N.M., The Shiva Foundation, 1997.

Cralle, Trevor. *Flinging Monkeys at the Coconuts*. Berkeley, Calif.: Ten Speed Press, 1993.

Dass, Ram. *Compassion in Action*. New York: Bell Tower, 1992.

Davidoff, Henry. *A World Treasury of Proverbs*. New York: Random House, 1946.

Dossey, M.D., Larry. *Healing Words: The Power of Prayer and the Practice of Medicine*. San Francisco: HarperSanFrancisco, 1993.

———— *Reinventing Medicine*. San Francisco: HarperSanFrancisco, 1999.

Duff, Kat. *The Alchemy of Illness*. New York: Pantheon Books, 1993.

Encarta Dictionary. New York: St. Martin's Press, 1999.

Feldman, Reynold, and Cynthia A. Voelke. *A World Treasury of Folk Wisdom*. San Francisco: HarperSanFrancisco, 1992.

Frank, Leonard Roy. *Random House Webster's Quotationary*. New York: Random House, 1999.

Frankl, Viktor E. *Man's Search for Meaning*. Boston: Beacon Press, 1992.

Friedman, Edwin H. *Friedman's Fables*. New York: Guilford Press, 1990.

Guralnik, David B., ed. *Webster's New World Dictionary of the American Language, 2d college ed.*, New York: Simon and Schuster, 1982.

Hanh, Thich Nhat. *Peace Is Every Step*. New York: Bantam, 1992.

Houghton, Patricia. *Cassell Book of Proverbs*. London: Cassell, 1992.

Keen, Sam. *Learning to Fly*. New York: Broadway Books, 1999.

Klein, Allen. *Quotations to Cheer You Up When the World Is Getting You Down*. New York: Wings Books, 1991.

———— *Up Words for Down Days*. New York: Gramercy Books, 1998.

Knaster, Mirka. *Discovering the Body's Wisdom*. New York: Bantam, 1996.

Lane, Deforia. *Music as Medicine*. Grand Rapids, Minn.: Zondervan, 1994.

Lerner, Max. *Wrestling with the Angel*. New York: Touchstone, 1990.

Lorde, Audre. *A Burst of Light*. Ithaca, N.Y.: Firebrand Books, 1988.

Lorie, Peter, and Manuela Dunn Mascetti, eds. *The Quotable Spirit*. Edison, N.J.: Castle Books, 1996.

Lown, Bernard. *The Lost Art of Healing*. Boston: Houghton Mifflin, 1996.

Macmillan Dictionary of Quotations. Edison, N.J.: Chartwell Books, 1989.

Maggio, Rosalie. *Quotations for the Soul*. Paramus, N.J.: Prentice Hall, 1997.

McNiff, Shaun. *Art as Medicine*. Boston: Shambhala, 1992.

Meider, Wolfgang. *Illuminating Wit, Inspiring Wisdom*. Paramus, N.J.: Prentice Hall Press, 1998.

———— *The Prentice-Hall Encyclopedia of World Proverbs*. New York: MFJ Books, 1986.

Microsoft Bookshelf 98 Reference Library. Microsoft Corporation, 1987-1997.

Moore, Thomas. *Care of the Soul*. New York: HarperCollins, 1992.

Original Self: Living with Paradox and Originality. New York: HarperCollins, 2000.

Moyers, Bill. *Healing and the Mind*. New York: Doubleday Main Street Books, 1993.

Naparstek, Belleruth. *Staying Well with Guided Imagery*. New York: Warner Books, 1994.

Oliver, Mary. *Dream Work*. New York: Atlantic Monthly Press, 1986.

Oman, Maggie, ed. *Prayers for Healing*. Berkeley, Calif.: Conari Press, 1997.

Oxford Dictionary of Quotations, 3rd ed. Oxford: Oxford University Press, 1979.

Phillips, Bob. *Book of Great Thoughts Funny Sayings*. Wheaton, Ill.: Tyndale House, 1993.

Potter, Peter. *615 Great Thinkers Tell You All about Death*. New Canaan, Conn.: William Mulvey, Inc., 1988.

Princeton Language Institute. *21st Century Dictionary of Quotations*. New York: Laurel Books, 1993.

Progoff, Ira. *At a Journal Workshop*. Los Angeles: J.P. Tarcher, 1992.

Quinn, Tracy. *Quotable Women of the 20th Century*. New York: Bill Adler Books, 1999.

Reader's Digest Quotable Quotes. Pleasantville, N.Y.: Reader's Digest, 1997.

Rechtschaffen, Stephan. *Timeshifting*. New York: Doubleday, 1997.

Remen, Rachel Naomi. *Kitchen Table Wisdom*. New York: Riverhead, 1996.

———— *My Grandfather's Blessings*. New York: Riverhead, 2000.

Roberts, Elizabeth, and Elias Amidon. *Honoring the Earth*. San Francisco: HarperSanFrancisco, 1993.

———— *Life Prayers*. San Francisco: HarperSanFrancisco, 1996.

Rosman, Steven M. *Jewish Healing Wisdom*. Northvale, N.J.: Jason Aronson, Inc., 1997.

Sacks, Oliver. *A Leg to Stand On*. New York: Touchstone Books, 1984.

Safransky, Sy. *Sunbeams: A Book of Quotations*. Berkeley, Calif.: North Atlantic Books, 1990.

Scheffler, Alex. *Let Sleeping Dogs Lie and Other Proverbs from around the World.* New York: Macmillan Children's Books, 1997.

Schneerson, Rabbi Mendel Menachem. *Toward a Meaningful Life: The Wisdom of the Rebbe.* New York: William Morrow and Company, 1995.

Setzer, Claudia. *Quotable Soul.* New York: John Wiley & Sons, 1994.

Shanahan, John M., ed. *The Most Brilliant Thoughts of All Time.* New York: Cliff Street Books, 1999.

Silverstein, Shel. *The Missing Piece Meets the Big O.* New York: Harper & Row, 1981.

Simpson, James B. *Contemporary Quotations.* New York: Harper Collins, 1997.

Sounds True. *Audiotapes for the inner life,* Boulder, Colo. 1-800-333-9185 or www.soundstrue.com.

Steindl-Rast, Brother David. *Gratefulness, The Heart of Prayer.* New York: Paulist Press, 1984.

Sylvia, Claire, and William Novak. *A Change of Heart.* Boston: Little, Brown & Company, 1997.

Templeton, John Marks. *Worldwide Laws of Life.* Randor, Pa.: Templeton Foundation Press, 1996.

White, David Manning, *Eternal Quest.* vol. 1. New York: Paragon House, 1991.

www.beliefnet.com

www.cybernation.com

www.healthjourneys.com

www.motivationalquotes.com

www.mythinglinks.org

www.quoteland.com

www.spiritualityhealth.com

Zerah, Aaron. *The Soul's Almanac.* New York: Tarcher/Putnam, 1998.

Permissions

■

THE AUTHOR AND publisher gratefully acknowledge the following for their permission to include excerpted material from previously copyrighted material:

Robert Bly for permission to use the untitled poem by Antonio Machado that appears with the word *Wisdom*. It is reprinted from *Times Alone: Selected Poems of Antonio Machado*, trans. Robert Bly (Middletown, Conn.: Wesleyan University Press, 1983).

The Charlotte Sheedy Literary Agency for permission to reprint the material from Audre Lorde, *A Burst of Light* (Ithaca, N.Y.: Firebrand Books, 1988).

The Guild for Psychological Studies Publishing House, San Francisco, Calif., for permission to reprint an untitled poem by Sadie Gregorie that appeared in *A Meditative Calendar November 25*.

Deforia Lane for permission to retell her story about Ginny.

Dan Millman for his version of the story about attitudes which originally appeared in *The Way of the Peaceful Warrior* (Emeryville, Calif.: H.J. Kramer, 1984).

Mary Oliver for "The Journey," from *Dream Work* (New York: Atlantic Monthly Press, 1986).

Steven Rosman for his version of the Mr. Yetzer story that appears with the word *Responsibility*.

Portions of the text for the words *Humor* and *Stories* originally appeared in articles by the author in *Spirituality & Health: The Soul/Body Connection* magazine (Spring and Fall, 2000).

Portions of the word *Journaling* originally appeared in an article by the author in *Intuition* magazine (*Intuition* did not use seasons or dates to identify its issues).

Portions of the text for the word *Life* originally appeared in an article by the author in *Forward Day by Day* (Cincinnati, Ohio: Forward Movement Publications, 1999).

If any permissions were inadvertently omitted, we ask your forgiveness and would like to hear from you so that the appropriate acknowledgments can be made in future editions.

About the Author

CAREN GOLDMAN SPECIALIZES in writing about spirituality, health, psychology, religion, and the arts. Over the last twenty-five years, hundreds of her freelance articles have appeared in national magazines including *New Age Journal, Natural Health, Yoga Journal, Spirituality & Health, Diabetes Self-Management, Intuition, Coping,* and *Forward Day-By-Day* as well as regional magazines and major metropolitan daily newspapers. She began her writing career as a news and features reporter at the *Cleveland Plain Dealer*. Caren leads retreats throughout the country and does Bridgebuilder™ conflict resolution consulting with churches, synagogues, and not-for-profit organizations. She and her husband, Ted Voorhees, live in Toledo, Ohio.

Caren can be contacted by e-mail at wordsforhealing@aol.com or via her Web site, www.carengoldman.com.